To: Jane

Remember to
Breathe Deep
and
Never, ever Lose Hope!

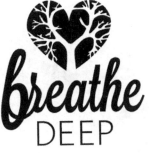

Blessings,
Kelly M.
Wever

2019

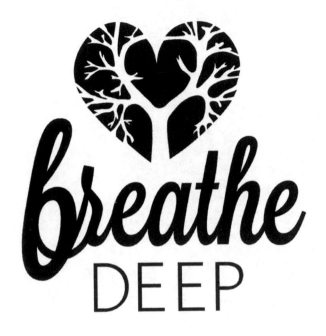

breathe DEEP

Life with Cystic Fibrosis and
Surviving a Double Lung Transplant

Kelly M. Wever

MILL CITY PRESS

Mill City Press, Inc.
2301 Lucien Way #415
Maitland, FL 32751
407.339.4217
www.millcitypress.net

© 2018 by Kelly M. Wever

Cover Design and Logo Design by Nichole Amberg

Edited by Stacy Doyle

Printed in the United States of America.

ISBN-13: 978-1-54565-088-2

Dedication

To my family and friends, for being my strength when I had none. And To God and my Donor, I owe my life to you.

Table of Contents

1
No Cure

There was no cure. There were no more treatments or medications that could help. No way of reversing the years of lung damage, scarring, infection, or inflammation. Both of my lungs were no longer able to adequately provide oxygen to the cells in my body. Carbon dioxide was building up in my bloodstream to a dangerous level. The excessive, forceful coughing was popping holes in my lungs and causing them to deflate. I could no longer live with my lungs. It was time for a double lung transplant, the last resort.

The year was 2010, and I had just celebrated my twenty-sixth birthday. I did not have the luxury of chasing my career goals or traveling the world in my twenties. Instead, I was contemplating a double lung transplant. I made an appointment for a lung transplant evaluation at a local hospital that was accredited for their lung transplant program. I would undergo a mountain of tests that would determine if I was a candidate for a transplant. This evaluation would essentially determine if I lived or died. The weight and importance of these tests were immense.

My transplant evaluation schedule was intense; it was physically, mentally, and emotionally exhausting. Four full days of tests and appointments. I struggled to even find the endurance for several days of testing. My days included: a ventilation-perfusion scan, a cardiac catheterization, a bone density screening, giving fifteen tubes of blood, numerous scans and x-rays, and meetings with the social worker, dietician, cardiothoracic surgeon, and the pulmonologists who specialize in transplant care.

After reviewing all of my tests, the doctors concluded I would potentially be a candidate for a double lung transplant, but not at this time. It was "too early." I was not sick enough. I needed to completely wear out the lungs I had. This was due to a shortage of lungs donated, and the average survival post-transplant was only five years. I needed to use my lungs as long as physically possible.

The doctors said my 30% lung function and functional status were still too high. The doctor estimated I would be ready for a transplant in one to two years. All I could do was fight to maintain my lung function. I had to be 100% compliant with medications, breathing treatments, chest physical therapies, and exercising. I remained diligent by undergoing transplant evaluations every six months. I was determined not to slip through the cracks and wait until it was too late. I could not afford to miss my window of opportunity for a transplant. I had to be sick enough to be listed, but not sick enough that I would not survive the surgery and recovery. It was a very fine line to walk.

Over the next three years, I returned for six more evaluations. Every time I wondered, "Is *this* the time I will get on the transplant wait list?" As time passed, with each evaluation, I had new concerns. I worried the longer I waited, the more likely the doctors would find something in my tests that would disqualify me from the transplant. I often prayed, "Will I ever receive a transplant?"

2

Rewind

L et me rewind and tell you how I got to this point. I was born with Cystic Fibrosis (CF). CF is a genetic, progressive disease that causes thick, sticky mucus and affects the lungs, digestive system, liver, sinuses, sweat glands, and reproductive system. CF causes repeated lung infections and limits the ability to breathe over time.

My normal life was the CF life. From the moment I was born, the doctors knew something was wrong. My abdomen was swollen and my colon was not functioning. The doctors were frequently measuring and re-measuring my abdomen, but the swelling did not go down.

I was taken to a children's hospital by ambulance with my Dad racing behind in his car. My mother was left at the adult hospital recovering from giving birth to me. Can you imagine your newborn baby being whisked away without knowing what was wrong? My parents were startled, scared, and shaken. They had no idea what was wrong with their baby girl or if I would survive this.

At the children's hospital, they performed gastrointestinal surgery on me, just a five-pound newborn infant. I had a meconium ileus, which meant that my intestines were stuck to my abdominal wall. The surgeons had to pry the intestines off of my abdominal wall. This resulted in the use of a colostomy for four weeks. A colostomy is when one end of the large intestine is brought through the abdominal wall and is stitched into place. This allowed my abdomen and intestines to heal properly leaving no long-time side effects from the surgery.

I was in the hospital for the first six weeks of my life. The doctors suspected it was CF. However, after being tested, the result came back negative. Maybe the meconium ileus was a fluke isolated occurrence the doctors reasoned. My parents were hopeful I would recover from the surgery and no further medical attention would be needed.

But, six months later, I weighed only six pounds. I was the same size as a newborn baby. I just did not grow. The pediatrician suspected I had "failure to thrive," a key identifier in CF babies. I was tested again, and this time the result was positive. I had Cystic Fibrosis. My parents were relieved to finally have an answer. The doctor prescribed pancreatic enzymes to aid the absorption of my food and that finally allowed me to gain weight. I had to take the pancreatic enzymes every single time I ate for the rest of my life. Thankfully, these enzymes did the trick, and I started growing immediately.

At this time, the life expectancy for a CF patient was only eighteen years old. A devastating and life-altering diagnosis for parents. My parents often wondered how to prolong that life expectancy for me. They believed if we stayed compliant to all the medical regimen prescribed, I could beat that statistic.

I had an older sister named Julie, who did not have CF. She was three years older and my parents pondered, "Should we treat Kelly the same as her older sister, or differently? Should we protect Kelly from germs and keep her out of pre-school?" So many questions and no right answer. My CF nurse encouraged my parents to let me do everything that my older sister was allowed to do. Not to treat me any differently. They were encouraged to give us an equal amount of attention, even with my illness requiring an excess amount of time and energy as parents. Naturally, my sister does recall being jealous because of the attention my disease attracted. She eventually grew to feel guilty over her jealousy, which is a complex emotion for any child. But, my parents did an extraordinary job at treating us fairly and making us both feel special.

My parents decided to send me to pre-school just like the other neighborhood kids. Then, on to public school where I was able to lead a normal childhood with only a few interruptions from my CF. My everyday regimen included dozens of pills throughout the day. Since I needed to take pancreatic enzymes before I ate, this required me to visit the school nurse every day before lunchtime. This was a big deal. I did not display any CF symptoms to my friends when I was young, but a trip to the nurse each day definitely set me apart from other children.

Another important part of my CF regimen was one breathing treatment and two chest physical therapies per day. At the time, only one breathing treatment medication was available to prevent lung infections. It thinned the sticky mucus, allowing the patient to remove the mucus before deadly bacteria could take hold. Unfortunately, many prescription drugs in the "pipeline" were being researched, but only one was accessible to patients.

My parents also performed a chest physical therapy called postural drainage every morning and evening for twenty minutes each. Postural drainage helps move mucus out of the lungs by using gravity and a clapping in certain areas on the chest. There are numerous positions used such as on your stomach, back, and sides, that all help to move the mucus out and unclog the airways allowing for easier breathing and less infections. Honestly, I never liked the postural drainage when I was young. But, as I got older and my disease progressed, I began to truly enjoy the postural drainage because it did alleviate symptoms and made me feel better. I would even fall asleep during the postural drainage due to the comfortable positioning and rhythmic clapping.

I saw the CF health care team consisting of doctors, nurses, dietitians, and social workers every two to three months. I performed pulmonary function tests at each appointment, which was terrifying as a little girl. The whole test was performed in a box similar to a phone booth. The forced expiratory volume in one second, or FEV1, was a test that involved taking in a deep breath and blowing it out as fast and hard as I could. At this time, my CF was considered mild and my lung function score, the FEV1, was about 80%.

Another test would require me to pant while cutting off the air supply to the booth. All of these tests were performed with nose clips on, ensuring I could not breathe through my nose. Some testing required the door to the booth to be closed; other tests were done with the door open. When the door was closed, I became very claustrophobic and deathly afraid I would get stuck in the booth. From that moment on, my grandpa came to my clinic visits just in case he ever needed to pry his little girl out of the box. Luckily, the claustrophobia fear subsided with age, but the breathing tests became more difficult to perform and the results had a real impact on my everyday life.

3

The Nature of the Beast

I had one short hospitalization at five years old as a routine "tune-up." This was when you were hospitalized and received several rounds of antibiotics to try and ward off any growth of deadly bacteria in the lungs. At this time, I was actually doing so well that my doctor tested me for CF again. It came back positive. My parents were just grateful that I was not experiencing any symptoms yet.

I had a significant drop in lung function when I was thirteen years old. My parents were terrified. To ensure that I did not miss any breathing treatments, medications, or chest physical therapies, they made my CF treatment regimen my household chores. They gave me a weekly allowance if I did not miss any treatments or medication. It was a great motivator for me as a teenager.

Unfortunately, my lungs were now home to Pseudomonas Aeruginosa, a deadly bacteria that 60% of CF patients accumulate. The bacteria can be picked up in kitchens, bathrooms, hot tubs, pools, sinks, and humidifiers: basically anywhere. Tragically, CF patients are unable to get rid of this bacteria on their own, and will likely never completely get rid of it once cultured. Luckily, the bacteria in my lungs was susceptible to intravenous antibiotics (IVs).

It was time for a hospitalization to fight the Pseudomonas Aeruginosa. Normal IVs in my arms would not work because the length of my IV treatment was so long. My veins would simply not hold up. The doctor told me they would have to place a peripherally inserted central catheter (PICC) line. Back then, a PICC line was a small catheter placed in the forearm and traveled up to the chest emptying into a large vessel. This enabled a patient to have extended IV therapy for weeks at a time.

I was in the seventh grade. Not an ideal time to hide a PICC line in your arm or make time for the hours of antibiotics my lungs needed. Plus, I was extremely scared to have a PICC line placed. Receiving my first PICC line was one of my absolute worst experiences. I was led to a small, closet-sized sterile room where the insertion would take place. Normally, patients can get their PICC line placed in the first or second try. I had to be a "unique" case.

The nurses tried again and again and again. Blood was flowing steadily and my complexion became paler. I nearly fainted multiple times. My Dad, who was there to hold my hand, even became faint and had to leave the room. It took three different nurses and seven tries to partially place the PICC in my arm. They never actually succeeded in correct placement.

They could only insert it about 20%. The PICC line was in my forearm and was supposed to go all the way to my elbow to the upper arm and towards the chest cavity. It was a long way for the IV antibiotics to travel to get to the chest cavity. We prayed the medications would work.

Fortunately, I was still able to receive the much-needed IV medications. I had an extreme regimen for these IV medicines and woke up really early in the morning for my parents to run the IV medicine before school. It would run for a couple hours in the mornings while I slept. Then, repeated again in the evenings.

The first few weeks it appeared the antibiotics were not working. My lung function was not responding. It took six weeks before my lungs responded to the hours and hours of IV antibiotics. My FEV1 numbers came back to baseline about 80%, and I was coughing less. I still had the Pseudomonas bacteria, but it was now minimized. Finally, my lung function had rebounded.

The biggest lesson my doctor taught me at this age was to continue to do my treatments and take all of my medications. Exercise every single day and stay compliant to the medical regimen. He made it clear that CF does not take any days off. No vacations, no holiday breaks, no Christmas vacation. CF was working against me every single day.

So, I remained extremely active in dance and gymnastics. When I got to high school cheerleading kept me active. But, despite my best efforts to keep my lungs healthy, I started coughing, which is a major side effect of CF. It was just small amounts at first and easily passed as a "cold" to strangers or distant friends.

Then, eventually, it became more frequent, coughing several times per hour. Next, I started having a productive cough where mucus would come out as I coughed. The mucus in my lungs was plugging my airways and my natural reaction was to cough out the infected mucus. It was now noticeable during class time and becoming harder to deny an illness. A fellow student in my Spanish class expressed concern to my teacher because of my coughing. She was genuinely worried about me.

At bedtime, the coughing was relentless. I would cough for hours trying to get to sleep. If I woke in the night, the coughing would start again. My parents would lay in their bed in agony listening to my coughing, and my mom would cry herself to sleep.

During my teen years, the Pseudomonas Aeruginosa bacteria that I cultured caused a permanent lung function decline and double lung infections. My FEV1 on my lung function testing declined to 60% through these years. Every morning I would take my morning pills and eat a high-calorie breakfast. I was always trying to gain weight. After that, it was time for my morning breathing treatments. A second inhaled antibiotic had come to market for patients. So I was on two nebulized medications twice per day. I took my pills independently at lunchtime and for a snack before cheerleading practice. I knew forgetting my pancreatic enzymes would result in a massive stomachache.

Once home from school, it was time for another breathing treatment and new chest physical therapy called, "The Vest." It was the new, improved version of postural drainage and cost about $10,000. It was a huge expense for my parents. "The Vest" inflated and shook at different designated frequencies and pressures. On the high pressure and high frequency settings, it would give me a productive cough. I had to wear this contraption for thirty minutes per day. Not fun for a teenage girl, but it beat doing the postural drainage with your parents.

I made it work. I planned my homework time during my "Vest" time. Killed two birds with one stone. After that, it was more pills before dinner, eating a high-calorie dinner, and off to bed early. I required way more sleep than my peers because my body was always fighting diseased lungs and working overtime.

Even with the challenges that my CF presented, I was determined to "go away" to college and have the ideal college experience. My parents were supportive of my decision, but also very scared. It is hard for any parent to see their child leave home, but if your child has a life-threatening illness, it is compounded with immense fear. They knew if I did not take care of myself the result would be catastrophic. They also knew that when I was sick, they were three hours away and in their mind, would not be able to get there quick.

My fear was having a roommate. I was afraid to live with a stranger. I did not want to perform breathing treatments or the chest physical therapy "Vest" in front of someone I didn't know. Not to mention, all the coughing, particularly the coughing I did at night, that could keep a roommate up.

Thankfully, my college allowed for single rooms in the dorm. I had a normal room just like everyone else but could have the privacy I needed for my treatments. I did my hospital "tune-ups" on all of my breaks from school. These "tune-ups" consisted of two weeks of IV antibiotics to try and maintain lung function. I had two "tune-ups" over the summer break and one over Christmas break.

There were a few instances when my CF did not adhere to my school schedule as I wished it would. My exacerbations were becoming more frequent, and when I developed any sort of cold or respiratory virus, it would turn into a bad double lung infection very quickly. My parents and sister became really worried and would make the three hour trip to pick me up from college. They would help me pack my bags and drive me back to my children's hospital three hours away. Each time they came to pick me up, they wondered how sick I really was and if I would get better.

The increase in exacerbations led the doctors to suggest a port-a-cath be implanted. The port-a-cath, or port for short, was a surgically implanted catheter threaded into one of the large central veins in my chest that empties into the heart. The port would replace PICC lines and peripheral IVs. It would allow IV antibiotics to be administered at college without a hospitalization or interruption in routine. But, even the word "port" was scary to me. I was not well-educated nor had I ever seen one, so I was very apprehensive to have one implanted.

Convinced the port was inevitable, I had one implanted. Turned out that receiving the port was one of the best decisions I have ever made. It made my life so much easier and reduced my stress during inpatient hospitalizations dramatically. No more PICC line insertions and less peripheral IV sticks.

Two months after having my port implanted, I started having extreme pain in my lower back. I had no injuries or explanation for the pain. I had several ultrasounds, scans, and biopsies. Much to my surprise, I had multiple kidney stones. The doctors could not figure out why I formed the kidney stones but reasoned it could have been from my medications. The doctors inserted a stent and said I had to wait for the kidney stones to pass on their own.

A couple months later, as I got ready for an evening out at a Christmas party, I started having severe lower back pain again. I had been looking forward to the party, and I had a new outfit all picked out to wear. The pain was worsening by the hour though, and now I found myself repeatedly trying to use the restroom. Then, an hour later, I was no longer able to walk, lay down, or use the restroom. I was in excruciating pain. My kidney stones had picked the wrong day to try and move out. I was supposed to be going to a Christmas party! How was it going to look if I canceled last minute? But, I had no choice, and I knew it was time to resign myself to the hospital.

I called the doctor and my parents drove me down to the hospital. The pain was unbearable. The emergency room confirmed it was the kidney stones. They were stuck in my urethra, causing the inability to use the restroom and extreme pain. The doctors performed a shock wave lithotripsy. This procedure sends high-energy shock waves to your kidneys and breaks up the kidney stones. Then, the stent allows the pieces of the kidney stones to pass over the next few days. The pain was constant, and no one knew how long it would take for the kidney stones to pass. So, I started on pain medication around the clock for three days until the last stone had passed.

During the college years, my FEV1 lung function score dropped to 45%. My lungs were very infected and scarred. There was irreversible damage done from the frequent and incessant infections. Despite the frequent hospital stays, infected lungs, and strict medical regimen, I still felt a sense of normalcy in my life. I was able to exercise, go to class, and hang out with my friends as I wished.

One Friday evening, I was out with my sorority sisters listening to live music at a local bar. My sorority sister introduced me to a fraternity boy who was there with a group of his friends. She said we would be a perfect match. It was the quintessential college meet cute. His name was Nathan, and he was wearing a blue striped collared shirt, worn jeans, and brown cowboy boots. A country boy in cowboy boots as my perfect match? It turns out she was right.

I never hid my CF from any new boyfriend, and Nathan was no exception. He had already commented on my frequent cough and there really was no hiding my illness. I told him about my CF on our second date. Surprisingly, he already knew. Word travels fast around the sorority house to the fraternity house. He did not know what CF really was or how it affected my everyday life though. He was blissfully ignorant of the seriousness of my disease and the mountains we would have to climb together. He had concerns about my CF and voiced those with his parents and close friends. They were a great sounding board for him. It was about a year before he realized the intensity, severity, and emotional drainage to love someone who has CF. In the end, he decided any time with me was better than no time, and he chose to love me regardless of the dark cloud that loomed over us. On the day of my college graduation, he got down on one knee and asked me to marry him. And I said "Yes."

4
Tying the Knot and Baby Fever

W e planned a warm summer wedding at sunset time. We invited all of our family and friends. On August 12, 2006, I got married to the love of my life, Nathan, in a church full of sunlight, family and friends, and bright gerbera daisies. We were just twenty-two and twenty-three years old respectively. We both knew our life would be a fast track. If we wanted to do something, not to wait. Life is short, especially if you have CF.

My parents were so proud to see me living my dreams and having a sense of normalcy in my life. They knew Nathan was the right man for me. He would be a protector, provider, and stand up for me. He was able to handle my CF and all the challenges that came with it. God had made him strong and healthy to take care of me. My new husband was just the motivation I needed to continue the hard fight against CF, stay compliant, and even dream of our future.

As a newlywed, the last thing you want to worry about is health insurance and affording your life-saving medications and equipment. But, this was the reality for us. I learned very quickly that my new insurance would not pay for a new version of "The Vest" or cover the entire cost of my expensive medications. I had to borrow a portable form of "The Vest" from my doctor's office or the sales representative when I needed it. Such a hassle!

Also, I was only allowed $10,000 for prescriptions drugs per calendar year. Within the first two months I met my medication maximum for the year. CF medications are ridiculously expensive. We worried about how to pay for my medications for the rest of the year. We lost sleep. We knew that without my medication, I would be in the hospital within days.

I talked with my healthcare team first. Were there any alternative, less expensive medications I could take instead? There were only two medications eligible to switch, all the rest were name-brand medications. There were no generics.

The pancreatic enzymes that I needed to take to eat totaled over twenty pills per day. The enzymes cost $3,000 per month. An astronomical expense that we could not afford to pay and this was just one of my medications! I was on ten prescription medications including two specialty medications, which were very costly.

I became very resourceful and creative. I called my doctor's office every couple of weeks asking for samples. If they had any in stock, I would rush down to the hospital and obtain any sample I could. Every little bit helped.

My family held fundraisers, enabling me to purchase remaining medications out-of-pocket. I price shopped around town for my other prescriptions. I was amazed at the price differences. One big box store charged $30 for a medication, while another private specialty pharmacy charged $120 for the exact same medication! I learned that price comparisons for my medications were crucial if I had to purchase medications from my wallet.

Just a few months after I got married, I was in for a routine tune-up hospitalization when my doctor asked me, "Do you and your husband want to have a baby?" I wanted more than anything to be a mother. My immediate answer was, "Yes." I was raised in a strong knit family and desperately wanted to have my own child. But, I also knew that the chances of having a healthy pregnancy was only 20%. Not good odds. I also had a decreasing lung function that was working against me. My doctor replied, "Don't wait."

So, at the young age of twenty-two, we started trying to have a baby. It was earlier than any of my peers, but I knew I had to live my life differently because of my CF. I read mountains of research on pregnancy in CF patients, joined blogs and chat rooms pertaining to the topic, and talked with my health-care team. My doctor advised me that I needed to have an FEV1 of at least 1 liter, or an FEV1 of 45% or higher, before I got pregnant.

I was just below this mark. I was determined to get to the 1 liter benchmark number on my lung function test. I started jogging and exercising more. I worked myself up to two miles of jogging. Such a huge feat, and it worked. I raised my lung function to 1 liter.

Our families were really nervous for me to attempt pregnancy and motherhood. They knew the physical strength needed and were really unsure if my body could handle it. We tried to get pregnant for almost two years. I was now twenty-four years old. I was tired of trying, tired of being stressed out over trying, and tired of being disappointed about a consistently negative pregnancy test result. I resigned myself to the fact that we would need an intrauterine insemination or in vitro fertilization, with my doctor's permission, in order to get pregnant. I was scared my doctor would not approve a procedure, thus leaving us with no child. I knew adoption was not an option either since I would not be able to pass any physical examinations.

Then, one Monday morning just before work, I took a pregnancy test. I had already decided it would be negative. But, I would head straight to work to distract myself from being disappointed and wondering if a baby was ever going to happen. Much to my delight and amazement, the test was positive. I could not believe it. I immediately performed two more tests-all positives. We were having a baby.

Our families were extremely supportive now and knew God would bring me through it. My pregnancy was surprisingly normal. My body knew just what to do despite my CF. My lung function actually increased, likely due to the pregnancy hormones. As I entered my third trimester though, breathing got difficult. I was winded when walking short distances. My baby was pressing up on my lungs, and this made my lung capacity suffer.

It was time to supplement my oxygen supply and start oxygen therapy. We needed to ensure my baby was receiving enough oxygen at all times and could grow. First, I started just wearing oxygen at night and when I exercised. Then, I started wearing the oxygen during the day too as my baby grew and my lungs became more pressed.

I was referred to a high-risk obstetrics specialist during my third trimester. His job was to determine if it was safer for me and the baby to have a vaginal birth or a cesarean surgery. My pulmonologist voted for the cesarean since the heavy breathing during labor would be difficult. The high-risk obstetrics specialist opted for the opposite. He said the vaginal birth would be a shorter recovery time and easier for me. But, it turned out that no doctor made the decision. God did. My baby was in a breech position and the only safe way to deliver a breech baby is a cesarean surgery. Decision made.

In May 2009, I had a healthy baby girl. We named her Molly Sue. She was the most perfect baby I had ever seen, and I got to call her my daughter. God entrusted me to raise this child, and I was so proud of my new Mom role. She was my new motivation to keep me at my best.

Unfortunately, the downturn of the economy led my husband to accept a new job twelve hours from home. Twelve hours from our family and friends, my doctors, and our entire support system. Our parents were crushed and worried about how I would handle full-time motherhood in a new state with my progressing CF.

We packed up all of our belongings and held our sweet four-week-old baby girl wondering what our new life was going to look like. We had to find a new home, new friends, establish new doctors, and adjust to parenthood all while balancing my CF regimen. Sadly, the demands of my new motherhood, a lack of sleep, living twelve hours from family support, and my taxing CF regimen took its toll. Within six months of having my daughter, my lung function dropped another 10%. My FEV1 was now hovering around 35%. When my daughter was seven months old, my doctor said, "It is time to think of a double lung transplant. There are no other options, and I know you have a daughter to raise."

5

The Downhill Slide

This brings me back to the beginning of my story. The results of the lung transplant evaluations truly had my life on the line. Plus, it was not just me anymore. I had a daughter to raise and she deserved to have a mother. My husband found a new job, and we were able to move back home after being away for eighteen months. We were ecstatic to be close to family and friends again. We knew we would need them during my transplant.

For three years, I underwent the transplant evaluations and had a real-life roller coaster ride. My whole family was invested in these transplant evaluations. We were all anxious, nervous, and distressed. We were on the roller coaster you do not want to ride and cannot escape.

My 35% lung function dropped to 30% and I started having fevers due to my infected CF sinuses. In December 2012, I had a very serious exacerbation. I was experiencing endless fevers, shortness of breath, and increased cough. I was admitted to the hospital. They performed a chest x-ray as usual.

However, the results were not the usual progression of CF in the lungs. The doctor found a nodule in my right lung. A million questions ran through my brain. What exactly is a nodule? Of course, I had heard the word "nodule" before but what is it made of? Was it cancerous? What kind of treatments does this call for? The doctors desperately wanted to know the composition of the nodule. They debated whether it was safe to go into my weakened lungs and take a biopsy of the nodule.

But, it was determined that the risks outweighed the benefits. I would simply have to live with this nodule not knowing what it was composed of, why it was there, how it would impact my CF, and no plan on how to get rid of it.

I was very scared so I did the only thing I could do. I prayed. I did a lot of praying. I was discharged from the hospital on IV antibiotics. Two weeks later, I returned for a CT scan of my right lung. We needed to see if the nodule had changed. Was it bigger? Was there another one starting to grow in my other lung? The CT scan was painless but nerve-wracking. I waited at home for my results.

A few hours later, my phone rang. It was my nurse coordinator. The doctor had reviewed my CT scan. He was astounded. The nodule was gone. Gone! I could not believe my ears. The doctor and nurse said they had no idea how it happened. Nodules do not just disappear in CF patients. But, I knew. God had faithfully answered my prayers. He had a plan for me.

In January 2013, I started on oxygen full-time. This was an ultimate low. I was extremely self-conscious about wearing oxygen. I felt sickly, undesirable, and loathed what the oxygen tube represented. I wanted to avoid going into public and meeting new people who asked too many questions. Questions I really did not want to answer. I did not want to have to explain the presence of the oxygen tube. I just wanted to go through the checkout lane at the grocery store without having to reveal my health history and prognosis to complete strangers. People were inclined to ask "what is wrong" when they see an oxygen tube on a young person.

Luckily, the oxygen did not bother my husband. He was more concerned about the self-consciousness I had over it than anything. He still saw me as his wife and the woman he loved. The oxygen tube did not stop that.

My daughter became so accustomed to the oxygen that she did not remember me before the oxygen. Mom with oxygen was her normal. She did not like that it prevented me from doing physical activities or outings with her like swimming or walking around the zoo. She was too young to be embarrassed by it.

The oxygen supply company gave me two portable tanks. Each tank lasted anywhere from one to two hours depending on how much oxygen I required at the time. The sicker I was, the more oxygen flow was needed. I could only be gone from my home up to four hours. If my oxygen was off for any period of time, my lips would turn blue. Consequently, I had anxiety attacks if my oxygen tanks got too low when I was away from home. I could not stay out of the house for any length of time. Working became extremely difficult, I was in and out of the hospital frequently, and now the oxygen was the last straw. I quit my part-time jobs.

One evening, I was feeling particularly down about my new life with oxygen. As I was tucking my daughter into bed, she stroked my cheeks and said, "Mama, I love you just the way you are—with your glasses, oxygen tube, and smile." It was exactly what I needed to hear. I realized she was the one I did not want to disappoint or to be embarrassed of my oxygen. Somehow my daughter always seemed to understand my unspoken struggles and knew exactly how to speak right to my heart.

In April 2013, I had another transplant evaluation. My lung function was now constantly below 25%. This was a substantial drop over three years. The doctors said it was finally time to get serious about the transplant. I was more than ready. I had been wearing oxygen full-time for four months and my quality of life was worse. My life now revolved around "How much oxygen do I have left in my tank" or "When are my next breathing treatments due?"

The doctors performed more in-depth tests before I was officially listed on the national waitlist. During this final phase of pre-tests, my bloodwork was checked to see if I had any antibodies present. I was not anticipating any red flags and that all would go smoothly. I was just ready to be on the list and to get on to my new life.

The result I received was a shock. As soon as the doctor came into the examination room, I knew something was wrong. The serious expression on his face, his formal posture, and soft tone of his voice told me that bad news was coming.

When the doctor started speaking, my concerns were validated. I knew he was about to drop a big bomb. "We found a very high level of antibodies in your blood work. This will make it extremely difficult to find a donor match for a transplant. Your antibody score is 99, which means only 1 out of 100 donors may be a match for you."

I could not comprehend what he was telling me. I had no indication I would have any antibodies. I didn't even know what an antibody was or its functions in the body, let alone how I accumulated so many of them.

The doctor went on to explain that antibodies are very common in the general public. I had about thirty antibodies in all, some of these running into very high percentages in the general public, making it even more difficult for me. My donor could not have any of the antibodies that I currently had or my body would recognize the new lungs as foreign and attack them. Rejection would be immediate and deadly.

My doctor went on, "the average wait for a double lung transplant is currently four months, but we fear your wait may be one to two years." One to two years?? Would I even live that long? My worst nightmare was coming true. I had been proactive for years. I came every six months for transplant evaluations. I was compliant. I did not want to be too late. I had other CF friends that waited too long to get on the transplant wait list and died while waiting for new lungs. I had been determined to not join that statistic. It was becoming my reality too. Was I going to die? The tears immediately started to flow.

6

The Wait

My wait officially began on June 21, 2013. I was twenty-nine years old and on the national wait list for a double lung transplant. Based on my lung function, my life expectancy was one year, and my wait time could be one to two years. I had no idea how this had become *my* life. Why was this the cards I was dealt? I had no idea what I was in store for, how long the wait would actually be, and if the transplant would ever come. There were so many questions and no answers. So, I prayed the transplant would happen much sooner than the doctors anticipated, and I would not get any sicker before a transplant came. I did not want my quality of life to become worse.

My family's support was simply amazing. They formed a team for me called "Breathe Deep." They provided support, meals, and held numerous fundraisers. The fundraisers included a carnival, pizza sales, garage sales, t-shirt sales, and a big fall family night out event with hundreds of people in attendance. My transplant social worker said that $25,000 would be needed to cover medical expenses, and my family raised enough money through fundraising that I never had to worry about my medical expenses. Such a gift when you need to channel your energy on surviving and not on insurance battles and medical costs.

I transitioned all my care to the transplant doctors at the hospital where I would be receiving the transplant. They would be able to manage all my prescriptions that way. Seems easy enough, however, the rapport I had with my former doctor was very strong. He knew my CF like the back of his hand. He was easily accessible for questions. When I felt sick, I had a direct contact line to him— a rarity in the field.

It was very hard to break ties and start seeing a new team of doctors. There were six pulmonologists, four pre-transplant nurses, a social worker, a dietician, two pharmacists, and several office staff that made up the transplant team. It was a struggle to learn the ways and habits of a brand new team. Each time I attended lung transplant clinic or was seen in-patient at the hospital, I seemed to see a different doctor. I felt like a fish out of water. I loved the idea of "six heads being better than one." However, the disadvantage was that it took me several years before I got to know each of the doctors treating me and for them to know me. It was especially tough during in-patient stays when I met the doctor treating me for the first time, and I was extremely sick.

My first inpatient hospital stay at my new hospital was unplanned, but surprisingly, comforting. It was for an exacerbation, a worsening cough, and an infection. It was time for IV antibiotics. Honestly, I did not have my expectations set very high after previous in-patient hospital experiences. I knew not to set the bar high considering what I had encountered at my former hospital.

After a short wait in the admitting office, I was taken to a private room on a floor dedicated to lung patients. My room was homey and spacious. All of the nurses knew exactly how to care for CF patients. My consistent, loud, sputum-producing coughs did not even make the nurse blink. I felt right at home. The respiratory staff came every four hours exactly as prescribed. I never had to request for respiratory to come. They showed up every time a breathing treatment was due. This alone was a welcome change and relief.

The doctors rounded at reasonable hours of the day. I was never awoken at 6am to see a doctor. The entire transplant team would visit me each day and assess my needs. I was able to pick what I wanted from a large menu. I had special snacks since I was a CF patient. My room was equipped with a large television with DVD player, and I was introduced to a movie closet. I had a Bose radio. Was this the Ritz? If you had to be in the hospital, this was the place to be! Needless to say, I was extremely satisfied with the care I received and the hospital itself.

Despite the exceptional care I received, taking every pill prescribed, doing every breathing treatment I could, exercising, and the endless support I had from family, my CF kept progressing. After all, that was the nature of the beast. CF is a progressive disease, and it just keeps getting worse, no matter how hard you fight it.

7

Deflated

My first real scare happened in February 2014. I had been listed for eight months. I noticed severe difficulty lying down at bedtime. I could not lay rested on my two pillows as normal. I was suffocating when I laid down. I compensated by buying a large wedge pillow, my daughter nicknamed, "the cheese pillow." The following days, I noticed more shortness of breath while walking, talking, and eating. I notified my nurse coordinator, and she told me to call if it continued or worsened.

The next day, I was walking to my car parked along a city street. It was a cold day and extremely windy. The wind literally took my breath away, and I could not get it back. I started walking backward trying to catch my breath. I was suffocating and could not get any air. My anxiety skyrocketed.

I hopped into my car and immediately dialed my nurse coordinator. I was so breathless that I could not even speak. The feeling of breathlessness and suffocation left me feeling completely unglued. I became more out of breath, which heightened my anxiety. I became more anxious the more breathless I became. It was a vicious cycle that I could not stop. I simply could not breathe.

I started to catch my breath, and I explained my symptoms to my nurse. My nurse was still not overly concerned since shortness of breath is such a common occurrence among transplant patients. Thanks to God, I was somehow able to drive myself home. I decided to just take an anxiety pill when I returned home. I really believed my lung function was worsening and my anxiety had taken over.

The following day I drove my daughter to the library. We were meeting her tutor there. I pulled into the handicap parking space. I tried to get as close to the door as possible. The short distance between my car and the front door of the library was going to leave me out of breath, and that made me anxious.

We walked towards the door, and I could feel myself struggling to breathe. I pushed forward towards the door while holding my daughter's hand. As soon as we walked through the doors, I immediately searched for a place to sit down. I was gasping for air. I could not walk any further. I sat down on a bench directly next to the front door. I could not speak or move. I was paralyzed and just trying to breathe.

I sat on that bench the entire tutoring session. How had I deteriorated this quickly? I could walk on the treadmill for thirty minutes with my oxygen pumping last week, but now, I could not even walk two minutes without gasping for air with my oxygen pumping on full volume. The thought of walking back out to my car was terrifying.

Something was wrong. I just knew it. I could not go on like this. I called my nurse for a third time requesting I be admitted. I needed to be checked out. I wanted to be seen by a doctor. This was not just my anxiety or my imagination.

I was admitted that evening. They ran blood tests, performed extra breathing treatments, and did chest physical therapy four times per day. My lungs were so filled with mucus the doctors were convinced this episode was nothing more than the typical exacerbation coupled with my anxiety. I believed these strong IV antibiotics would soon kick in, and I would reap the benefits.

After a couple days in the hospital, I still was not breathing any easier. The doctors were preparing for me to go home the following day and setting up home infusion therapy for IV antibiotics at home. I was trying to trust my new doctors. I did not know what the CF progression looked like, how it presented, how quickly one's lung function could drop, or the importance of severe breathlessness.

The following day, I was scheduled to be discharged. I was wheeled to the pulmonary function laboratory where they could gauge exactly how far my lung function had dropped before I went home. I got into the telephone-like booth, put on my nose clips, and was instructed to take in one big breath and blow out as fast as I could for about ten seconds.

I could not take a deep breath. I felt like I had no air in my lungs and was suffocating, again. The results were a huge blow. My FEV1 was only 14%. The lowest number I had ever seen.

My previous FEV1 had been 19%. I did not have 5% lung function to lose. I swallowed back the tears as they wheeled me to my chest x-ray.

I went into the cold, dark x-ray room. Luckily, I was still in the wheelchair because I would not have been able to walk from the doorway to the x-ray machine and stand there to perform the test. I stood with my chest facing the x-ray board wondering how I was going to take in a deep breath and hold for one to two seconds, which was the normal protocol for a chest x-ray. I struggled to hold my breath for even a single second. Somehow the technician managed to get the images needed. I was wheeled outside of the x-ray room and waited for the transport employee to wheel me back upstairs to my hospital bed.

I had only been sitting there for two minutes when two x-ray technicians came rushing over to me. "Have you been experiencing shortness of breath?" one of them said looking at me with worry. "Yes for about one week," I confirmed. They both nodded and assured me I would be taken back to my room shortly.

I have been receiving chest x-rays ever since I can remember, and I have never had an experience quite like that or had a technician come and speak to me directly after. Never had an x-ray technician seemed so worried. Oh dear Lord, what was on that x-ray? My anxiety went through the roof and my mind was racing. They clearly identified something in my x-ray that was abnormal. What was wrong? What could it be?

I was whisked back to my room on the thirteenth floor. I had the last room on the left, which was my favorite room on the floor. It was bigger and had lots of windows bringing in lots of light. It had a view of a city park, and I could see an ice rink with skaters gliding around breathing the fresh air and enjoying life.

I peered out the window and watched the ice skaters wishing all this would just go away. Wishing I had never been born with CF and wondering "Why *me*, Lord?" My nurse came rushing in and said, "You have a pneumothorax." She explained that a pneumothorax was when air enters your chest cavity and causes the lung to collapse. She placed a breathing mask on my face. It had a bag attached to it that inflated as I breathed out. Well, if I was not anxious when this bomb was dropped, I was definitely anxious now. The mask was supposed to help try to re-inflate my lung. Fat chance! I couldn't even breathe with this contraption on, let alone take in a deep enough breath for this thing to be beneficial. I started to cry.

Now, I had to break the news to my family. I knew they would be worried about me, which I hated. I pulled out my phone and started to text my family members. I could not speak. I was too breathless, nervous, scared, and overwhelmed. I told them the x-ray had shown a pneumothorax, and I was waiting to hear what the doctors wanted to do. All of my family immediately got in the car and flew down to the hospital. My parents and sister were trying to make it to the hospital before I was taken away for any procedures to heal the pneumothorax.

Nathan was able to get to the hospital quickly since he worked just minutes away. I could see the worry on his face as soon as I saw him. I squeezed his hand and gave him a hug. I was too breathless to speak.

I had many hospital experiences under my belt, and have never seen the hospital staff move as quickly as they did that day. There was no "hurry up and wait." It was quite startling to see everyone bustling in and out of my room. A surgeon came in immediately and explained the severity of my pneumothorax. "I am going to have to insert a chest tube," he said. What's a chest tube? Will that hurt? How long will I have this chest tube?

The surgeon explained that the chest tube would allow the chest cavity to release the trapped air and allow the lung to re-inflate. This could give me some immediate relief in my breathing. Yes, please! More people bustled through the door: nurses, technicians, and aides. The chest tube was going to be placed right where I was, at my bedside. I slipped on a gown and hopped in bed. This was happening right now. My parents and sister had not even arrived at the hospital yet. I was not being put to sleep or given anesthesia. It was "go time." 3, 2, 1...

I rolled onto my side and the surgeon numbed and cleaned the area. I gripped one nurse's hand and braced myself for the pain. This was going to hurt. Immediately upon the entry through my skin, I heard it. *Whoosh.* The air that was stuck in my chest cavity was coming out. After the air was released, there was a strange sensation. The surgeon inserted the chest tube in my side and up into my chest cavity. I had some immediate relief. Breathing was easier already, and I was less anxious.

The chest tube remained there for several days. It attached to a small box that collected blood and drainage that came out through the chest tube. I disliked the chest tube, and it made sleeping especially difficult, but, within three days my lung was 95% re-inflated. I was not able to do a breathing test to check my FEV1 for several months in fear it might collapse the lung again. Regardless, I went home being able to walk again and sleep comfortably.

8

Dazed, Confused, and Desensitized

hree months later, there was another blow— a new low. I
was thirty years old, and had been on the transplant wait
list for eleven months when I started waking up in the middle of
the night with severe headaches. One particular night, my headache was so severe that I was confused, dizzy, and my brain
was "foggy." During the day, I had trouble thinking. I could
not perform simple math and pay our bills. I could not think
straight no matter how hard I focused. This had never happened
before. I chalked it up to being overly tired. I walked to the
bathroom and was not able to catch my breath. I had no idea
what was happening. It was time to call the doctor. Something
was wrong yet again.

I called the emergency line for the transplant team. I was
admitted to the hospital on a Saturday evening, and the doctors
ran many tests, including a CT scan. The fear was a blood clot
in my lungs or maybe a severe exacerbation. Just last week, I

was able to walk on the treadmill for thirty minutes, and today, I could not even walk ten feet to the bathroom. I had a constant, worsening headache with no relief from pain relievers. The doctor ordered a blood gas test for the next day at 6:00 a.m. when the levels are optimal.

At 6am the next morning, a therapist came in to draw the level. These needle sticks are more painful than the usual. The blood has to come from the artery on the back of your wrist. Ouch. To top it off, at 6 a.m., my dehydrated arteries are not easily accessible. The therapist tried twice to access my artery. When she failed, she sought a second therapist. This therapist tried five times. Finally, on that fifth try, there was a blood return. Hallelujah! Now, it was time to sit and wait for the results.

A few hours later, the doctor came in for his rounds. He had the results. My blood gas was seventy-five. It was considered a critical level. A normal blood gas range is thirty to forty-five. The air exchange in my lungs was no longer performing the way it should. My lungs could no longer carry carbon dioxide out of the bloodstream; thus, resulted in a buildup of carbon dioxide. The only way to decrease the carbon dioxide in my bloodstream was to wear a machine at night that would release the carbon dioxide as I slept. This would be a slow process to lower the carbon dioxide.

All day, I had a severe headache, and it caused me to be nauseous and confused. That evening the respiratory therapist wheeled an average volume assured pressure support, or AVAPS, into my room. The AVAPS machine was essentially a non-invasive ventilator. Another new life-altering medical machinery for me to adjust to.

My sister stayed the night with me to help ease my anxiety of this new medical device I needed to wear every time I slept. I had no clue how in the world I would sleep with this thing wrapped around my head, suctioned to my face, and covering my nose and mouth. I could not even relax just thinking about wearing it, let alone sleeping with it on.

The therapist was extremely patient with helping me get used to the machine. I left the TV on all night. I needed a distraction from the loud noise the machine made and from the mask I had to wear. It controlled my breathing. I had to change the way I breathed when falling asleep. My breathing was always very fast, along with my heartbeat—working overtime. Eventually, I was able to drift off to sleep with my new machine.

In addition to my new sleeping companion, I was missing my daughter immensely. It was Mother's Day and the last place I wanted to be was the hospital. I wanted to be making memories with my daughter or at the very least, just hug her and tuck her into bed on Mother's Day. We were able to speak and see each other over Facetime, but my heart still hurt.

It took months before I slept comfortably with the AVAPS machine. But, after some time, I became to depend on the AVAPS. I could not imagine sleeping without it. I went from being afraid of wearing it and wondering how in the heck I would sleep with it to not wanting to go one night without it. It helped me sleep better and gave me more energy the next day. My lungs were rested with the AVAPS, and it helped me keep living.

Due to my decline and requirement for an AVAPS machine to survive, the doctors suggested desensitization treatments. The desensitization process had three components, which included: chemotherapy IV medication, pheresis treatments three times per week, and an infusion called intravenous immunoglobulin (IVIG). The pheresis treatments were a blood filtering process that eliminated the portion in my blood that held my antibodies. This desensitization process had the potential to decrease my antibodies and thus, increase my chances of finding a donor match. However, due to the intensity of the treatments and low success rate, the desensitization treatments were a gamble and not the preferred route. Additionally, after transplant, there were more complications. My two options were to try the desensitization process or wait for the perfect donor match while my health declines. There was no easy road.

I was really torn on whether I should go through with the desensitization process or not. In a perfect world, I would sit and wait for my perfect donor match to be found. But, in reality, my health was declining and time was not on my side. My family came up with a prayer and asked hundreds of our friends to recite the same prayer at the same time on the same day. It was called a prayer storm and we would storm the heavens with our prayers. God would hear us!

"Dear Lord,
We ask for your many blessings tonight on behalf of Kelly as she has reached a critical stage in her fight against CF. Lord, I ask right NOW for you to do

something mighty and powerful in Kelly. Her journey has come to a narrow path facing many challenges with much uncertainty. Please give her caregivers the wisdom to make the best decisions for her that provide a path of least resistance to her new lungs. We ask you give Kelly courage, strength, love, and a sense of peace in the coming days. We are anxious for something powerful and miraculous to occur and we are relying on YOU! We gather in unity pleading that you reward Kelly's spirit and determination with a chance to Breathe Deep! Amen."

Hundreds of family and friends recited this prayer during a beautiful sunset at seven in the evening. I had a sense of peace and without hesitation I decided to try the desensitization process. I spent fourteen days in the hospital. My husband would come visit me on his lunch hours and bring me food that would far surpass anything on my hospital lunch tray. My mom, sister, aunts, and uncles would bring me dinners, desserts, and entire baskets of treats for me to munch on throughout my hospital stay.

I knew this hospital stay would be especially long and tough on Molly. Being away from her mom for fourteen days was going to be really difficult. I made an activity chart full of fun outings to go on and friends for her to see. Each day a different family member or friend took her on a planned adventure. I don't think she wanted mom to come home!

The fourteen days were more tiring than I could have ever imagined. The pheresis treatments were performed every other day and left me completely drained. I could hardly hold my eyes open after six in the evening, and my legs felt like jelly. I also had side effects and unforeseen circumstances during each treatment. In the first treatment, I blacked out and in the next, I had horrible leg cramps. Then, the pheresis filtering machine stopped working in the middle of the treatment. It was a weekend and no one was available to help fix the machine. The technician had to call a 1-800 number on the side of the machine. Perfect. My anxiety level became higher and higher every minute I had to sit in the hospital bed with a large portion of my blood sitting next to me in the machine. The last thing I needed was to add a blood transfusion to the list. Blood transfusions can give you antibodies!

I had horrible luck with these treatments and an increased amount of anxiety with each one. They also left me with little energy for my CF treatments and regimen. But, it paid off. The initial results showed my antibodies were wiped in half! I was ecstatic. All the needle sticks, powerful medications, and blood filtering treatments were paying off. We kept going.

I was able to come home and undergo outpatient IVIG infusions and continue pheresis treatments three times per week to remove my antibodies. My family rotated chauffeur scheduling for me as I was too tired to drive after the pheresis treatments or infusions. During my first IVIG infusion, I had a horrendous reaction. I become extremely flushed, tired, and began shaking uncontrollably. The entire stretcher I was laying on was shaking

45

violently. After a large dose of another medication to counteract the reaction, the IVIG was stopped. I was so hopeful the desensitization would continue to work, but without IVIG, the odds did not look good.

It was a Saturday and my home health nurse came over for a routine flush of my central line that was placed for my pheresis treatments. My nurse pulled back on my line and expected a blood return. There was none. Only air. She immediately clamped the line, and I headed for the Emergency Room. This was not good. I was determined to fix the problem and have them place a new central line if needed. I had another pheresis treatment on Monday that I had to attend if I was going to continue to decrease my antibodies.

After several tests in the ER, the doctors figured out my central line had cracked. An anomaly that had apparently never ever happened before. I was the "unique case" once again. This crack in the line caused air to get into my lung, causing a blood clot in my lung. This was extremely serious and life-threatening. My family was really afraid for me and for my life. I was driven by ambulance at midnight to a special ICU where I was closely monitored. Nathan slept in the waiting room not wanting to be too far from me. This was my first time in the ICU. I joked to my family and nurses that I was camping since there was no private restroom, no privacy, and no sleep!

The next day, my central line was safely removed, and I immediately started blood thinner medication. Within a few months, the blood thinner medication resolved the blood clot. However, the doctors ended the desensitization treatments fearing I may not survive another blood clot and the IVIG reaction was so severe. My antibodies rebounded quicker than the blink of an eye and came back with a vengeance. My antibody numbers were even higher now than before we started the desensitization process. I made it through yet another hoop, but now it was back to waiting for my needle in the haystack.

9

The Heartaches

The hardest part of every single hospital stay was being away from my daughter. Hands down. When she was younger, I was able to slide by the first few days of a hospital stay by letting her spend a few nights at Grandma's house. But, eventually she would ask, "Wait, where's Mama?" Tears would flow down her sweet cheeks when I would tell her via Facetime that I was in the hospital. There are no words to describe the heartache I would feel in those moments. I missed her so deeply. Keeping her routine as normal as possible helped, but it was not enough.

My daughter loved coming to see me at the hospital, and we tried to make it as fun as possible. We would snuggle up in my hospital bed and watch her favorite videos or watch a movie she enjoyed. I would save her favorite snacks from my hospital meal tray. I tried to have a special prize from the gift shop.

When I was young, at the children's hospital, my doctors always called my hospital stays, "parties." We would have an endless supply of snacks, movies, and games to play in between breathing treatments, medications, and chest physical therapies. I tried to bring this same "party" atmosphere when my daughter came to visit me.

When it was time for her to leave, that was the worst part of my hospital stays. It was so hard for her to go back home and go about everyday life without her mama. Go to sleep without her bedtime tuck-in. Go back to school and concentrate. Do homework with someone other than Mama. Being separated from her made both of us not only stronger as individuals, but we were truly able to enjoy each other's company so much more when I came home. That first "welcome home" hug was always the best feeling in the world.

Luckily, Nathan was able to visit me often at the hospital, and we were able to stay connected just by seeing each other. He viewed my long hospital stays as something we had to do, a non-negotiable, and there was no reason to be down and out because of it. He became very good at dealing internally with his emotions and the chance of losing me. He rarely expressed his worries with me because he assumed I had enough issues going on. He was trying to protect me.

At home, Nathan was able to maintain some normalcy and keep busy. He could easily take his mind off of the negative thoughts. But, when I was in the hospital, he was forced to deal with my declining health. His faith helped carry him through the difficult part of my hospital stays when my disease was pushed to the forefront of our lives. He believed God would not put him in a situation that he could not handle.

My parents and sister also tried to bottle up and conceal their worries in an effort to keep my spirits up. My sister was an amazing advocate for me during every hospital stay. She would speak up to the doctors and nurses ensuring I had the best care possible. My past doctor mentioned that my positive attitude and sunny disposition were the reasons I had made it so far and lived far beyond the statistic. My family believed that too.

I had been on the waiting list, waiting by the phone for over two years. Surely my time was coming soon—right? I was constantly hit with one problem after the next on a downhill spiral. I was on the roller coaster from Hell.

My CF was now affecting all facets of my life in a major way. The breathing treatments got longer and longer due to my breathlessness and the need for frequent breaks. I needed more oxygen, lessening my time spent out of the house. I constantly had torn chest muscles and ligaments due to the repeated, forceful coughing making it difficult to walk. Hospital stays became the norm and the hospital felt like my "home away from home." All the staff knew me. My days and weeks were planned around my hospital stays. The emotional, social, physical, and spiritual ups and downs were nothing short of exhausting on all levels.

The emotions were the hardest part of the roller coaster ride. I have always been optimistic, and tried to see life as the "glass is half-full." It is in my DNA. But, that was tested so many times now. I was losing myself and my positive outlook.

I vowed to myself that while CF was able to control many aspects of my life and how I spend my time, it would not change my personality.

My emotional lows were always during times of physical lows and struggles. I had moments of weakness asking God, "Why? Why do I have to suffer this?" During each physical blow, I was forced to think about dying and not receiving the new lungs that I so desperately needed and wanted. What would dying look like? Would it be sudden or slow and painful? I honestly did not know what end-of-life looks like for CF patients, and the "what if" scenarios took a toll on me.

I wanted some control back. So, to decrease my negative thinking, I made myself do the things that I truly liked to do. Things I used to enjoy. Sounds simple, doesn't it? But, how often did I actually do what I like to do? Once per week? Once per month? I made a list of things I truly enjoyed and how often I wanted to do them. This was my new goal and something positive on which to focus. I found peace in the slowing down. I enjoyed the simple, little things much more. Watching a sunset, playing fetch with my dog, a good meal, and snuggling by the fire. I was allowed to slow down and discern what my priorities were. I simply did not have the physical strength, endurance, or enough oxygen tanks to do it all.

My social life was largely impacted. It was not about going out at night. Simply, going out to eat with my husband or going to a birthday party with my daughter. I had to intentionally skip big family Christmas gatherings, baby showers, or get-togethers with sorority sisters. I had to avoid crowds, especially during flu season.

I tried to be extra careful in public, bringing my hand sanitizer with me wherever I went. I knew that catching a cold did not mean being uncomfortable for a couple days. But rather trouble breathing, constant coughing, not sleeping, a long hospital stay, hundreds of doses of IV antibiotics to endure, and most importantly, being away from my daughter. Knowing the consequences of catching a virus led me to really shelter my outings. One gathering was not worth the result of weeks of recovery.

Only the very top priorities would get done. I had to maximize the time I had. I could not attend all the activities expected of me and be the perfect wife and mother that I longed to be. I experienced a lot of guilt over this. I wanted to attend charity events and parties as my husband's plus one. I wanted to take my daughter to Girl Scout camp and to the zoo. I felt overwhelming guilt because I couldn't attend. I was not the wife or mother I wanted to be, and the guilt was crushing.

I came to rely heavily on my parents, sister, and aunts to babysit my daughter and chauffeur her to all her lessons and meetings. Every weekend, my sister and her husband would take Molly for a fun outing and give me a much needed break. Molly also spent several nights per week at my parents. She loved spending the night with her Gigi and Papa!

My entire social support system of family and friends was nothing short of amazing. They made every attempt to lighten my load while I was in the hospital or sick in bed by doing our household chores, cutting our grass, cooking us dinner, and constantly providing physical and emotional support to me and Nathan. I thank God every day for the amazing people he put in my life.

Physically, I depleted so much energy just coughing all day long. I was so breathless that I could no longer do my laundry, cook meals, walk to the mailbox, go grocery shopping, or perform other daily chores. After a round of IV antibiotics, I was breathing easier, walking without difficulty, and able to get out of the house easier; but, household chores were still a huge feat. The question was always— "How long will I feel the effects of these antibiotics?" Sometimes they would last two to four months before I needed more IV antibiotics. Other times it was only two to four weeks.

My physical limitations meant one outing per day. The repercussions when overexerting myself and doing more were downright scary. If I overexerted, by the end of the day, I had difficulty breathing. Just sitting and breathing. I would skip dinner, struggle to walk to my bedroom, crawl into bed, and put on my AVAPS. Finally, relief would set in and my lungs could rest.

I had to sleep for at least twelve to fourteen hours in order for me to function the next day. Often, I would still be short on energy anyways. I was out of steam before my day even got started and would have to return to bed to rest. Many mornings, by the time I had gotten dressed, my daughter ready, off to school, performed all my breathing treatments, and ate breakfast, I was tired enough to go crawl back into bed. I napped every single day. I simply could not make it through the day without one. I would have serious repercussions if I tried to stay up and not let my lungs rest.

Spiritually, I yearned for a stronger faith and a closer relationship with God. I envied the people who were bold with their faith and always seemed closer to God. Like they had a direct line to God in their prayers, but I stumbled not knowing exactly what to say or how to ask what I really wanted. I wanted desperately to find a church home. So, in the midst of all of my roller coasters, I knew it was time to really devote myself to a church, read God's word, and deepen my relationship with Christ. It was the only way to find peace with my life and health challenges.

A friend told me about her church. It was the denomination I wanted, and the perfect location for me. God gave me the perfect window of opportunity to find a church. I loved the Pastor's messages. They spoke right to me and made a difference in my everyday modern life. The church met people right where they were spiritually and there were no judgments. You were able to be yourself, as imperfect as I was. I felt like I fit right in, oxygen and all.

I started helping in the church office once per week. I wanted to help and feel as if I had a purpose. It gave me one. It gave me something to keep my mind occupied and my hands busy. It also allowed me to deepen my relationships within the church. My new friends provided me with support and prayers every time I was hospitalized and needed desperately to hear them. I gained a deeper understanding of God's intentions for me and learned about patience and true faith.

10
Deflated...Again

I had a major turn for the worse in October 2016. By this time, I had been on the transplant wait list three years and four months, and I was thirty-two years old. I was far beyond the anticipated transplant wait time and surpassed the life expectancy. I was definitely on borrowed time. While the average wait time was only four months for most patients, I knew I was in for one or two years. However, I never dreamed I would be sitting there over three years later still struggling. My turn was overdue and I wondered if my transplant would ever happen. Was there a point to getting my hopes up or my family's hopes up?

My left lung had collapsed yet again. Another chest tube was inserted, but it did not work. This time the lung would not re-inflate because it was too infected and scarred. The hole in my lung that caused the collapse would not heal. The constant coughing kept the hole from closing. The doctors discussed a very risky surgery with unknown outcomes. The surgery would involve adhering or gluing, if you will, my lung to the chest cavity wall. This would help heal the hole in my lung and help for the immediate future, but create more complications during transplant, if a transplant ever came. During transplant, the surgeon would have to pry the glued lungs off the chest cavity wall potentially damaging it and causing excessive bleeding. After the surgery, I would have to be on the AVAPS machine for several days to let my lungs rest. This would mean laying in bed for several days and losing any muscle strength or weight I had left on me.

The doctor did not know if I would recover from a lung surgery. My doctor said he was very nervous for this surgery, but it may be our only option. My doctor had never been nervous about my outcome before. My lungs were just too sick, scarred, inflamed, and infected. My lungs wanted to just shrivel up and not fully inflate.

For the first time, I really questioned if I was going to die. It was questionable if I would make it through the surgery. If I did make it through surgery, could I make it through the recovery? Then, if I made it to transplant, the transplant would be much harder.

I prayed more. It was the only thing I could do in this powerless situation. I received a phone call from my pastor. He prayed with me over the phone, and what he said really stuck with me. He said, "God would stick his finger in my lung and plug the hole that would not heal." I visualized this constantly in my head. Within two days, the hole healed. After two weeks of the hole in my lung, God had healed my lung. No more surgery needed. My doctors left my hospital bedside scratching their heads. A "unique case" once again.

The hole had healed, but my lung did not re-inflate because it was too diseased. With the hole healed, I relished in the idea of going home. This had been my longest hospital stay ever. I went in on Halloween and came home the day before Thanksgiving. I had missed out on so much, and the aching in my heart to see my daughter was excruciating. Also, now, I had to live with a collapsed lung on top of an extremely low function and somehow still maintain normalcy in my life and my family's lives.

I had to take action. If I could not advocate for myself, then who would? The United Network for Organ Sharing, or UNOS, manages the nation's organ transplant system. UNOS controls the national transplant wait list. Patients are ranked by an allocation score. This score consists of approximately twenty factors, which includes: age, diagnosis, blood chemistry levels, oxygen dependency, and functional status. The allocation score does not have an allowance for antibody levels. My antibodies were the primary reason I had not received any offers for lungs; however, the antibodies were not even taken into account when the lungs were allocated to patients. How could that be?

My doctor petitioned to the UNOS board because of my "unique case." He said it was a long shot, but worth a try. The doctor's plea was denied. Luckily, just as God had planned, the national UNOS conference was being held in just one week in my city. What were the chances? I had many family members eager to help me present my "unique case" to them. We were desperate to make them understand that I did not have the time to wait for that 1% chance any longer. If I waited until I was in complete respiratory failure and on a ventilator, I would not have the time to wait for my "needle-in-a-haystack" lungs. I would die waiting for a transplant.

I was contacted by a local television news channel who was covering the UNOS conference in town. The reporter wanted to explore a personal story with transplant and how viewers could help. He came out to my house and interviewed my family and me. I was extremely nervous to tell my story to the world, but I knew the importance of organ donation awareness. It saves lives. After hearing my personal story and connection to organ transplant, friends and complete strangers signed up as organ donors.

My family and I wrote letters to the UNOS board to ensure they heard our plea. A second doctor sent the board a request on my behalf. He asked for an exception due to my current pneumothorax and high antibody levels making me a "sensitized" patient. This time, we were heard. I was granted an exception in December 2016, which allowed me to receive a donor match even if my score was not at the top of the list. I prayed and prayed my suffering was coming to an end and for a donor match to be found.

11

The Ultimate Low

January 3, 2017, was a new low. I performed blood work, a chest x-ray, pulmonary function test, and saw the doctor. I sensed another bomb drop as soon as the doctor entered the room. My doctor's outlook on my survival odds had changed. The hope of a transplant was quickly diminishing. My absolute worst fear was realized. Up until this day, my medical team had remained optimistic I would make it to transplant. However, with my multiple pneumothoraces, antibodies score, and current collapsed lung, the odds were stacked against me. I had so much to live for, and I felt it slipping away.

On the drive home, I cried the entire way. Then, I reminded myself that my God was the only true healer. There was still a chance. I was alive and breathing, and that was enough. Nonetheless, I was heartbroken that night and turned to scripture. I messaged an associate pastor at my church who immediately responded with several scriptures for me to read and study. He encouraged me to pray boldly. I knew God heard my cries, but praying boldly was my last option.

God continued to lay the groundwork and weave together all the necessary pieces for me. I had an unwanted insurance change on January 1, which left me with the frustrating process of obtaining approval for the transplant yet again. It took three weeks before I had a letter in hand stating a transplant would be covered by the insurance.

Additionally, I had mild cold symptoms requiring IV antibiotics. It was rare these days to start IV antibiotics at home and administer them the entire two weeks. But, this was the case, and I was able to manage my cold symptoms and improve without a hospitalization. I was able to spend time with my family.

It was my 33rd birthday and I had a birthday celebration allowing me to spend time with friends. The next evening, I went to worship with family and saw church friends. I listened to the Pastor's words, which I so deeply needed to hear that evening. I was tired, worn out, and acutely aware my days were limited.

12

The Call

On Sunday, January 29th, I put my daughter to bed at 8:30 p.m. It was just like any other night. We read a bible story, prayed for new lungs, and snuggled in bed. I fell asleep around 10:00 p.m. and stirred slightly when the house phone rang. Then, my cell phone next to my bed rang.

It was 10:30 p.m. Not a time that I receive calls. I rolled over expecting a wrong number on the phone. It said "unknown." I decided that I better answer it regardless of my sleepy mind and the hassle of disconnecting my AVAPS machine. My husband was still sound asleep.

Immediately after I said, "Hello," and heard my nurse's voice, I knew. My time had finally come. Prayers answered. My heart leaped out of my chest! I hopped out of bed and put on my oxygen. My nurse stated, "We may have a match for you. Do not get your hopes up yet though. Everything looks good on paper, but we have not seen the lungs yet. Go ahead and get ready and come down to the hospital."

I was trying to remember how to breathe. I was nervous, desperate, and hopeful. This was the first call I had ever received of a potential match for me. I desperately needed this match to work. It was my only chance.

I nudged my husband to wake up. In disbelief, I said, "It's time! They may have a match for me!" His sleepy face was in complete shock, the same as mine. Was this actually happening? Was this a dream? Pinch me!

I called my family. I woke my mother from a deep sleep. When she saw the caller ID on her cell phone, she knew it could not be good news. Calling late at night either meant I was struggling to breath and needed to be taken to the hospital at once, or Molly was sick and I needed her help. I blurted out, "They might have lungs for me!" My mom was completely stunned and scared to death. She scrambled around trying to figure out how to get dressed and put herself into the car. She was completely numb and could not get her brain to think. After sharing with my sister, she was confident and said, "This is it, Kelly!"

After throwing on my clothes and shoes, I went to my daughter's room. She was sound asleep. Her bedside lamp was on, and she looked so peaceful and angelic. I had run a million scenarios in my mind over the last three years about when I received my call. Where would I be? How would I react when I received my call? But, most importantly, how would I tell Molly? Will she be scared that she would never see me again? Will it be hard for me to give her that "last" hug goodbye? Will I be able to walk out the door not knowing if I was coming home?

I sat down on her bed and rubbed her back until she was just awake enough. I told her that the doctor had called, and I may be getting new lungs. I had to go to the hospital. I had left her notes and little prizes for each day I was in the hospital. I would be sleeping for the first few days, but we could Facetime after that. Grandpa and Grandma were going to take good care of her. She simply smiled and said, "Ok, Mama" and drifted right back to sleep. Just what I needed to have the courage to head to the hospital. God gave me the complete peace and strength I needed. I knew that in order to keep living and to see her grow up, the transplant was the only way.

13
Last Moments

As we drove to the hospital, my breathing was accelerated and my heartbeat was racing. I texted family and close friends, said silent prayers, and tried to remain calm. As we drove the winding, country roads to get to the highway, my husband was as nervous as I had ever seen him. He looked up into the expansive, starry night sky and saw a beautiful shooting star. He knew it was a sign from God that all would be right again.

It was now January 30th, the day my life would be forever changed. When I got to the hospital, I was honestly expecting a small army to descend upon me and get me hooked to machines, take dozens of tubes of blood, perform my last breathing treatments, give me an update on the status of the lungs, sign a stack of forms, and the list goes on. Instead, I was ushered to a floor that frankly did not seem to even know I was coming, and didn't have a room ready.

After waiting at the nurse's station, I was ushered into a shared room that was ninety degrees inside. It was like a sauna. I like to keep my hospital room nice and frigid, and I had not shared a hospital room since I was five years old. The harmful bacteria my lungs carried always ensured a single room.

I had the bed by the window and the heater pumped out hot air like no tomorrow. After a few hours of laying around and sweating, I finally received word. My surgery, which was previously scheduled for 4:00 a.m., was pushed back to 9:00 a.m. Darn! I was ready to get this show on the road and get out of this hot room. The attending doctor did not know if the lungs were viable yet. My nurse reasoned that the lungs may be coming from far away since the surgery was pushed back several hours. Turns out, she was right. The lungs were coming all the way from sunny California; a long way from Missouri. Very fitting as my nickname my whole life has been "Miss Sunshine."

The hours crawled by and exhaustion took over. I dozed off. Around 7:00 a.m., I was ushered down to the pre-surgery waiting area to sit in a "parking spot" area. More waiting and wondering. At last, at 9:00 a.m., I was given the green light! The lungs were viable and the surgery was set for 10:30 a.m. I wanted to scream! "Praise God!" This was happening! All the waiting, the tears, the collapsed lungs, the hospital stays, the treatments, the pills, and the disappointments were coming to an end. There was light at the end of the tunnel. Oh, to be able to take a deep breath. Imagine the possibilities!

The next hour consisted of several "see you later" conversations and hugs, not goodbyes. Lots of hugs, kisses, prayers, and laughs about my family driving a hundred miles per hour on the highway to get there before I headed into surgery. They made it with five minutes to spare. I told my family that as soon as I woke up I wanted to know, "How am I doing?" and "How is Molly?" My mom and I were both surprisingly calm and ready for the surgery. An anomaly because we are never the calm ones. We giggled as my husband asked, "Why am I the nervous one?"

I headed into the operating room at around 10:00 a.m. I had a whole church staff praying for me at the exact time I was rolled into surgery. The surgeon was upbeat, positive, and very friendly. He made me feel completely comfortable. He remarked how I did not seem nervous. I said, "My lungs are not going to last much longer, Doc." The operating room was as I expected. Large, sterile, white, and chilly. It was a welcome retreat compared to my shared sauna room upstairs.

The team of doctors, nurses, respiratory therapists, and anesthesiologists all prepped me and were ready to roll. They took away the oxygen tube and had me breathe into a mask as they prepared my line for general anesthesia. I was staring up at the bright light on the ceiling reciting Exodus 14:14 over and over in the head, "The Lord will fight for you; you need only to be still," "The Lord will fight for you; you need only to be still," "The Lord will fight for you; you need only to be still." That was the very last thing I remember as Kelly Wever, Cystic Fibrosis patient with respiratory failure, oxygen dependency, FEV1 of 14%, positive for Pseudomonas Aeruginosa,

Aspergillus Niger, and Staphylococcus Aureus." That girl was gone forever. New lungs meant a new life. My old life was being traded for a new one.

14

Double Lung Transplant

As surgery was underway, my family congregated in a small surgery waiting room playing cards, nervously chatting, and piddling on their electronic devices. Nathan does not recall how he spent the next six hours of waiting and recalled being in a daze. My family said there were lots of tears flowing and hugs given. Every hour they would anxiously await an update on how I was doing in surgery.

My sister started alerting extended family and friends on social media. Asking for prayers and sharing in our rejoicing. My sister started a "Caring Bridge" website so people could follow my progress frequently. Her posts are the best recollection of the next nine days as she wrote them in real time.

January 30, 2017: Kelly Starts Her Journey to Breathe Deep

12:30 p.m. Surgery has begun to transplant two new donor lungs.

January 30, 2017: First Update

2:22 pm ~ Just received a call from the surgical team... Everything is going well so far. They are about to transplant her new "right" lung.

January 30, 2017: It's A Miracle!

5:02 p.m. ~ The surgeon just came to the waiting room with an update. Kelly is doing great! Both lungs were successfully transplanted and are (in his exact words) "Working Perfect!" We were all in tears of joy and could not believe what we were hearing. Kelly will be moved to ICU within the hour and will remain there for the next few days. The Dr. is hopeful that she will only be on the ventilator through mid-day tomorrow.

Already making great strides towards breathing deep.

January 30, 2017: She's in Recovery

7:00 p.m. ~ I have never experienced so many emotions at once... The doctors are amazed at her progress already. We were able to hold her hand, kiss her arm, and best of all she could hear us! She even gave us a thumbs up! It was the most rewarding and truly remarkable moment. She will remain on the ventilator, and currently has four chest tubes to monitor the drainage, but everything is looking great! Thank you again for the prayers and thoughts, please keep them coming Kelly's way!

I awoke in the intensive care unit. I was alive!! Thank you, God! I had made it through surgery in just six hours and kept unconscious for six more hours so my new lungs could acclimate. I was attached to a ventilator, which was performing my breathing for me. The ventilator was letting my body rest and the new lungs adjust to their new home. I had anticipated that I would be very confused and forgetful of where I was when I awoke in the ICU. But, much to my surprise, I knew exactly where I was, what my body had just undergone, and just how important these next 24-48 hours would be. I was only awake a few minutes before I was pulled back into unconsciousness.

70

January 31, 2017: First Night Success

We are happy to say... No new changes, which is great! No complications her first night. Kelly was able to write a couple notes about her faith in God- "God's Work" and "God is Good." This morning the testing will begin to see how the lungs are responding. If all goes well, Kelly will come off the ventilator today. Please send prayers and more notes... She will love reading all of the prayers and well wishes when she is able.

The bounding excitement deep in my veins did not keep me under for long. I knew that I had survived my double lung transplant, and I was ready to fight my way through this upcoming battle of recovery. I awoke and squeezed my husband's hands. A few family members came into the room to see me awake for the first time. I motioned to my family that I wanted to write. I needed to convey the pure joy that I was feeling. All that kept running through my mind was "God is Good" and "Thank you Lord for this miracle." I have to say that my writing was relatively decent considering all the sedatives and pain-killers I was on!

In the middle of the night, all the lights in the intensive care unit were off and no one was sitting in my room when I awoke. I was not scared, but I wanted reassurance from the nurse that I was alright. Seeing as I could not speak or reach for my call light to my nurse, I clapped my hands over and over. The logical form of seeking attention, right?! My nurse came in, "Tomorrow is a big day. Try to get some sleep." That was just the reassurance I needed as I fell back into the unconscious.

January 31, 2017: Breathing Deep

Kelly received her bronchoscopy this morning and everything looks good. Very little bleeding. Her stats all look great. After the round of tests... We are proud to say, Kelly took her first unassisted breath at 9:10 am. She has officially been off the ventilator for over an hour and doing well. She is very tired and uncomfortable, but not in any pain. Which we are grateful for! Her Dr said, "if you must have a double lung transplant, this is how to do it" and pointed at Kelly.

As Nathan said, (referring to her first breath) "This was an amazing moment and one I will never forget."

Today was a good day. Her stats continued to stay consistent and they were able to remove her SWAN line early this afternoon and her femoral line roughly thirty minutes ago. She is currently laying flat to make sure the artery clots properly. Throughout the day, her pain levels were varied and she had bouts of nausea, but overall she was comfortable. They did start her on additional pain medications, to stay ahead of as much pain as possible (and a med to combat any additional nausea).

There were several firsts accomplished today also...

- *Kelly was able to get out of bed and sit in her chair for roughly two hours.*

- *She stood next to her bed and was able to take small steps in place- 50 to be exact.*

- *She had ice cubes for lunch and jello (2 flavors- cherry AND lime) with a cup of apple juice for dinner - yum!*

- *I brushed her hair... It's the little things we love!*

The morning came quickly and it was a big day. First, it was a quick bedside bronchoscopy by my pulmonologist to check on the new lungs. The doctor gave the green light, and the respiratory staff was there to attempt to wean me off the ventilator. It was about to get real. It was time to see just how well my new lungs were working. Were these new lungs going to do the job? Over the course of the next thirty minutes, the respiratory therapist allowed me to start taking breaths that eventually got to a normal breathing rate. Then, just like that, the ventilator tube was gone.

Next, it was time to see if I could go for an hour on my own. I tried staying very calm and concentrating only on my breathing. I did not want to have to go back on the ventilator. I made it through the hour with flying colors. The first breathing test was a success. These new lungs were working on their own! I was given oxygen with the hopes of decreasing its flow each day. Oh, the possibilities of life with no oxygen. How glorious that sounded!

One of the most intriguing moments of the day was when the huge team of medical students and doctors would congregate outside my ICU "stall" and discuss my progress and plan. Was I supposed to be listening? I wanted to ask, "Can you talk louder out there?" I felt like I was eavesdropping on my own treatment plan. Should I be listening or pretending to be sleep? The doctors were truly amazing, and I loved learning from them.

I was still very sleepy, but I did sit up in the chair for quite some time and took several steps standing in place. Another small accomplishment! It felt good to stretch my legs and get out of bed. I quickly wore out though. Baby steps.

January 31, 2017: Fill her Room with Happiness

Please help make Kelly's day (and decorate her room for the coming weeks) by sending a card. You are able to send an e-card through the hospital's website. These cards are printed out and hand delivered to her room. Please include a wish, prayer, or bible verse. Our goal is to have a hundred cards delivered to her room. This small gesture (that is free and takes less than a minute) will mean the world to Kelly. Thank You for your help!

My sister asked friends and family via social media to send e-cards to me through the hospital's website. I received over two hundred e-cards! It was so touching. Each day, my sister would gather the cards and read every single one of them to me. The staff would bring in a fresh stack of e-cards every day that were inspirational and full of love. A true highlight of my day. They said I had set the record for most e-cards!

15

Recovery

February 1, 2017: Day 2 Post Op

Another Day, More Accomplishments!

Kelly was able to have her radial line and catheter removed. She does have a small leak in her right lung, but the doctors are still saying everything is looking good. There is not a lot of concern with the leak, just something they will monitor. Her blood sugars have been elevated throughout the day and currently receiving insulin injections. The medical team is relating that to her steroid medications and have hopes that her levels will return to normal range.

Kelly made great strides with PT today. With Nathan behind her (with a chair in case) and my mom and

I at her side with her therapist, she amazed all of us and walked three hundred ft!! She made a steady stroll around the ICU. This girl is unbelievable! She didn't become winded at all, the toughest part was the pain surrounding her incision as she walked. That is currently the one thing she is battling... The pain. However, you would never know. All of the staff already loves her and appreciates her positive spirits and beautiful smile!

She's already their favorite :)

By the end of the day, Kelly graduated from the ICU and was moved to the cardiothoracic floor. She also started on solid foods today. For those who don't know Kelly personally, she loves to eat! You would never know this petite, 5'1" sweetie can pack away some food. We can't wait to start bringing her some of her favorites.

Overall, another great day. Our family would like to thank everyone again. All of the calls, texts, emails, posts, etc. have been so heartwarming and greatly appreciated. We hope that you will also take a moment to say a prayer for the donor family. Words cannot express our gratitude for their selfless decision to donate their loved one's organs. They saved the life of my sister and we will be forever thankful!

I was up and walking around the intensive care unit with therapists, IV poles, an oxygen tank, a backup wheelchair, a walker... and a partridge in a pear tree. All this while in my hospital gown. It was quite the show. Walking for the first time was not as painful as anticipated due to the benefits of pain medicine. At this point, I had four chest tubes, two on the right and two on the left, an intrajugular IV in my neck, IV in the groin, port accessed, EKG cords, etc. I was ready to start removing all these darn tubes and quickly learned a sense of humor was crucial.

I graduated to a normal hospital room, got my catheter removed, and the IV in my groin pulled out. Making solid progress! I was elated to have a private room with a door and a bathroom. Privacy! Oh, the simple pleasures in life.

It was quite an adjustment changing from the ICU to the cardiothoracic surgery floor. In the ICU, the nurses pretty much lived in my room and checked on me several times throughout the hour. On the cardiothoracic surgery floor, nurses came in about every three to four hours, unless I called on them. I suppose that is just par for the course, but it led me to need family at all times.

February 2, 2017: 100 is a Great Number - Day 3 Post Op

Kelly had another day of accomplishments.

- *No oxygen was needed all day! Her O2 stayed stable at 100!!*

- *Her anterior chest tubes were removed, only the posterior ones remain.*

- *She got out of bed more freely today and spent a lot of the day in her chair.*

- *And the top accomplishment of the day- Kelly walked a thousand ft with just a standby assist. She was talking and walking, something most of us take for granted. But this small thing is huge for Kelly. Not only was she able to walk and talk... She did it without oxygen and her stats were good.*

They will continue to watch the air leak and her blood sugars, as they are still high. But it was a good day! We are so proud of Kelly and her daily accomplishments. She is working hard to get home and spend time with Molly.

They have a bucket list of things to do with her new lungs!

My oxygen was slowly getting weaned. Within four days of having my new lungs, I was breathing on 100% room air and no longer required oxygen. I repeat, NO oxygen! Thank you, Lord! This was a life-changer. I had lived with oxygen for over four years and my life revolved around it. There were no tanks to tote around. I felt twenty pounds lighter. I had the possibility of being able to be gone from my house all day long. This was all new territory.

Pure amazement I experienced as I watched the oxygen saturation machine read "100%." I could not remember the last time I had no oxygen and my oxygen saturation levels were 100%. It had to be when I was a little girl.

I had two chest tubes removed today. This made life much easier. Getting out of bed and sleeping were still difficult though. I could not get comfortable while sleeping with the chest tubes in and my sides were so sore after their removal. My sides would "ooze," if I laid on my sides, which was my preferred method of sleeping. The nurse changed these chest tube dressings every few hours to keep them clean and dry.

I liked having someone spend the night each night. My husband stayed with me the first week, then he had to get back to work. My mother was watching my daughter who had caught a cold and pink eye. So, she was unable to stay with me and my aunt stepped up. Thank goodness for family. They were able to help me when I was at my weakest point.

I received several yummy take-out meals, desserts, and special treats. I never watched my blood sugar before. It was a foreign concept to me. Sweet treats now meant insulin shots. Luckily, the doctors anticipated a decrease in my blood sugar levels as my medication dosages decreased over time.

February 3, 2017: Day 4 Post Op

Today was a little harder for Kelly. The pain is really setting in and the swelling is uncomfortable. They are now giving her additional pain medications routinely, no longer as needed. We are hoping this will provide her with more relief during the day. She was pretty wiped out today... The doctors wanted her to sleep as much as possible. She couldn't catch a rest break, so I quickly remedied that when I arrived late this morning. As Kelly calls me, the door nazi, I ensured no one bothered her when it wasn't necessary. Routine is key- do everything needed at one time and then she would receive rest breaks for nearly three hours at a time. No more vitals... and then fifteen minutes later a med pass... and then ten minutes later forgetting to take one of the vitals... No more, this girl is on a routine now. I was not going to write about this, but Kelly insisted everyone know how ridiculous I am, no really she thought it was great! And thought people would chuckle. Love her and her positive spirit, always thinking about others!

The air leak is still there and being monitored, while her blood sugars are already looking better.

Even though the pain is high, she pushed through it during rehab today. Our amazing Kelly walked at .5 on the treadmill for THIRTY minutes!!! No oxygen!!! Her O2 stats never dropped below 95. We cannot describe how proud we are of her. Nate got her some new Beats by Dre (she's hip now) for hitting her walking goals.

Kelly started the education portion of her new life. Her new medications will be lifelong, and the next part is learning all about them. She has always been compliant with her CF routines, but she will be trading in the old routines for new ones. And we are so happy to have this routine instead!

I have been reading her all of the cards throughout the past few days. So far, she has received two hundred and two! We definitely met my original goal of a hundred. But she loves them, so keep them coming! It is so good to see her smile... And the messages have been so kind and uplifting.

We try not to make her laugh, but this video my aunt created to celebrate her new lungs, made Kelly laugh out loud (we made sure she hit her pain pump). Our dad with a mullet, her brother-in-law in a dress jumping out of balloons, and Nathan spiking the punch have been some fan favorites.

The pain was really starting to set in now and extra help getting up and moving was crucial. Each day, I walked longer and further. I got up to thirty minute intervals and increased speed each day. The respiratory therapist brought the treadmill right into my room each day. Perfect!

The sleep deprivation was really hitting me hard. It was one of my biggest hurdles in the hospital. I have always required a lot of sleep, and receiving new lungs did not change that fact. Plus, I had a new anti-rejection medication that affected my sleep now. This medication was due at 11:00 p.m. each night and kept me awake most of the night. If I did fall asleep, I experienced wild, vivid dreams. I was told it was a side effect from the medication. I was beginning to look like a walking zombie though from the sleep deprivation, and it was really affecting my energy level during the day.

My pharmacist came by today and taught me all about my new medications. These medications would be taken for the rest of my life. There were lots of side effects, but they were keeping me alive. The benefits outweigh the risks and side effects. Without these medications, my chance of rejection was a guaranteed 100%. I quickly absorbed the importance of my medications and knew my life was now going to revolve around these new pills and specific times I needed to take them: exactly every twelve hours. It was overwhelming, but I tried to remember that my "old" CF medications would be gone. No more breathing treatments. No more antibiotics. It was such a strange concept for me to wrap my mind around. A new routine to learn and adapt to.

February 4, 2017: Day 5 Post Op

Today the pain was better. Instead of being at an eight (out of ten) she was around a four or five. The consistency with the pain meds is helping to stay ahead of the pain. The doctor removed her right posterior chest tube... Only one chest tube left! With one side "tube free" she was able to lie on her side to find more comfort while sleeping. And yes, I was there all day again and she slept for several hours throughout the day.

After the removal of her chest tube, she had another chest X-ray. Everything looked good. She does have extra swelling (possibly a little fluid) on her left upper chest. Something her doctor will continue to watch. Hopefully, her last chest tube will come out on Monday, as well as her PICC line.

With the absence of the physical therapy team on the weekends, we were her therapists. She walked twenty-five minutes without oxygen around the 7th floor. She had a quicker pace than the previous days. She did great!

Many have asked how Molly is doing... Well, besides coming down with pink eye, she is doing great! She has been Facetiming Kelly and getting her visits in that way. She is happier than anything.

Kelly also experienced The Salon (me & my aunt) today. Hair washed and styled and a foot massage- may not be what she is used to at a spa, but she was quite pleased. And there is a nifty invention... A shower cap with shampoo in it. You throw in the microwave to warm it and then put it on your head and go! It works perfectly when you can't get your neck wet. She loved it! It's her second hair wash this week... I might be making a career change.

Thanks again for all of the support!

The highlight of my day was talking with Molly over Facetime. I had not told her I was no longer wearing oxygen. When she saw me she exclaimed, "Mom, your tube is gone!" My eyes welled with tears. What an incredible feeling! My daughter had not seen me without oxygen, as my real self, since she was four years old. I am not sure she really even remembered me without oxygen.

On the weekend, the respiratory therapists are off, so it was up to me to exercise. My sister helped me walk around the hallways at the hospital. I walked in my gown, footie socks, and a messy bun, but I didn't care! I proudly walked with no oxygen, ready to take my new lungs for a test drive. I exited my room to commence my hospital walk around the hallways when I saw my doctor. He watched me and smiled. I did not see him smile often, so it was something I will always remember. I can't imagine how rewarding it is to see your patient breathing easy for the first time; to give them a second chance at living.

I got pampered today, too. My muscles were sore from lying in bed so much. So, my aunt treated me to foot and back massages. My sister utilized my "free" shower cap from my hospital room. It turned out to be an amazing contraption. A method to wash your hair without using water! The simple pleasures in life...having clean hair.

Nathan got things done around the house today. He rounded up all my medical equipment and sent me a picture asking, "Can we get rid of all this now?" The photo was an entire dining table full of equipment that I needed to breathe and simply, survive. Now, I did not need any of it! How mind boggling!

February 5, 2017; One Week Since The Call– Day 6 Post Op

Today was a good day. Kelly's pain remained around a four, which is good! She was able to make several FaceTime visits in between naps. Her pain is mainly along her incision and in the swollen area of her upper chest. They have been keeping heating pads on her upper chest to ease the pain.

Late this morning, her final chest tube was removed. She had another chest X-ray and no news to report. She is officially tube free!!! The only uncomfortable thing remaining is the PICC line, which will hopefully be removed tomorrow. Kelly still has drainage after the removal of her chest tubes, but it is common and will just continue to keep her dressings changed. She will have chest X-rays frequently to make sure there are no changes.

Her sugars have been good... No insulin has been needed. She even had cheesecake and cherry pie. Today, Kelly and I walked for about twenty minutes around the orthopedic floor. There was literally no one there, even the nurse's station was closed. So it was nice not to have lots of people... fewer germs!

She looked the best today... Her color was good, her feet are less swollen, and she was more rested. Things are heading in the right direction. Tomorrow we will have an education class to teach us about Kelly's new routine and medications.

We are eager to learn and help with her new journey.

Slowly, I was able to get rid of all the chest tubes and IVs. I got the large IV in my neck removed and my last chest tube. Man, that felt good to have those gone. I could now move freely and sleep as I wish. My scar from the surgery, called a "clam-shell," goes from one side of my chest all the way to the other side. It was healing well. My fourteen inch incision was sealed with a super glue, if you will, that fell off in three weeks.

The swelling in my chest was really starting to worry me and becoming more uncomfortable. My breast tissue had been moved around during surgery and resulted in painful bruising and swelling. I was not sure if ice or heat would help. I was desperate for relief, so I tried both. My nurse aide was constantly on the hunt for them for me and even searched multiple floors to find them. So, there I was with heat packs medically taped to my chest when any visitors came by. Pretty comical! Not what I expected to receive with new lungs.

February 6, 2017: 1st Week Complete- Day 7 Post Op

What a whirlwind this week has been... From the initial phone call, to the surgery, and finally the first week of recovery. Kelly and our family have experienced so many emotions- disbelief to hope, fear to happiness, and of course anxiety but most of all encouragement. We have been so encouraged by the progress Kelly has continued to make and by the support and love of our family and friends. Kelly says she is blessed to have all of you in her life, but I say we are blessed to have her in ours. She has shown us that with strength, determination, and faith, miracles can happen. I am lucky to call her my best friend and sister.

After just one week, Kelly's doctors are already planning her discharge. She will be home before this weekend, less than two weeks post-op. She is still battling the pain, especially in her upper chest. She will continue on her pain meds for up to four weeks, and taper into a routine Tylenol dose until the pain is completely gone. Everything is starting to heal though and looks good. She walked for thirty minutes on the treadmill today. And O2 was stable! No oxygen has been needed for any exercise this week... Which is incredible!

We met with Kelly's post-transplant coordinator today. It was very informative. The reality is setting in, her new routine will be strict, but well worth it. She will go to the hospital Monday through Friday for the next three months. Her visits will consist of daily pulmonary rehab, twice a week blood work, and chest x-rays, once a week PFTs and doctor visits. She will need a bronchoscopy once a month as well. After the first three months, everything will taper off and become a maintenance program. It will eventually only be visits every six months. Her medication regimen will also be very scheduled. Depending on the rate of rejection (it is common to have rejection), her meds can be changed up to twice a week to control the level of rejection. She will remain on anti-rejection medications forever.

The future's so bright for Kelly. We are so happy for her to start living life to its fullest!

My new nurse coordinator outlined my new routine today. It was strict. It was going to keep me very busy. I had to devote all my weekdays to recovery and fighting through the physical pain. I was not going to go home and put my feet up until I felt better. In addition to the normal wife and mother responsibilities, now I added five days a week for three months of rehabilitation and tests to my schedule.

I was so used to my old CF routine that it was hard to envision a new routine. Any trip to the hospital in the past simply exhausted me, and I was looking at doing it five days per week now. Plus, I was going to have to depend on family to drive me around for six weeks. Not driving was going to be a huge loss of independence. How was I going to manage this new life?

My biggest concern at that moment was my lack of coughing. I was not coughing, not at all. I didn't even have the occasional "normal" person cough. I brought this up to my doctor and he pointed out, "You don't need to cough anymore." I had coughed my whole life, and in recent years, hours and hours per day. A day without coughing, what a miracle!

I anticipated breathing deep would be my greatest accomplishment with new lungs, but the lack of coughing was. It was startling how a lack of coughing drastically improved my life. I regained literally hours per day by not coughing and an entire day's worth of energy to be used elsewhere. The possibilities were endless!

February 7, 2017: Day 8 Post Op

Kelly experienced some side effect from the pain med-ication (most likely). She had blurred vision in her left eye and had pretty severe headaches. The headaches in return caused her to be nauseous and become ill. She has decided to stop taking the pain medications and switched to Tylenol only yesterday. She is hoping the Tylenol will be enough... But she will always have pain medications available, to help on days when the pain is unbearable.

My pain medication was reduced from an IV to oral medi-cation. Unfortunately, I learned very quickly that if I didn't eat a large snack or meal at the same time I took the pain medica-tion I paid for it. Nausea, vomiting, and a pounding headache would immediately follow. I had to either handle the effects of the pain medication or experience the pain. Not a fun choice.

It had been eight days since my double lung transplant and the doctors were planning my discharge already! All my chest tubes were out, and the leak in my lung had healed. Things were healing nicely, but I was in so much pain that it was scary to imagine being at home with no button to call when I needed to beckon for help.

I had become dependent on the nursing staff and the doctors' expertise. I felt safe at the hospital. What if these lungs stopped working all of a sudden? What if my chest continued to swell? What if something was wrong and I don't know it? What if I had a bad side effect to a medication? Was my insurance going to allow me to receive all these expensive, specialty medications by the time I go home? The list went on.

I knew my house chores and responsibilities waited at home for me. There was sure to be a pile of laundry to do, a week's worth of mail to go through, bills to pay, dishes to wash, and meals to prepare. I did not feel good. My emotions were all over the place due to my steroid medication. I was in pain and overwhelmed. I wanted to bury myself under the covers until I felt 100%.

February 8, 2017: Day 9 Post Op

After her visit today with the doctors, we will get the official release date. We have hopes that it will be today! Though it seems to be so fast, the doctors say her progress is great and want to get her out of the hospital to avoid unnecessary germs. As of last night, she is now feeling confident and ready to come home. She's ready to sleep in her own bed and hug Miss Molly!

We will keep you posted. Please continue to follow Kelly's journey...

This was the day. After a night of mentally preparing myself for my release from the hospital, I was ready. It was time to leave the hospital. I had received wings and now it was time to see if I could fly. All my major fears were put to rest before I left the hospital. I took comfort in knowing the hospital was just a short drive away if I had any emergencies. My nurse coordinator made sure all my medications were delivered bedside and in hand before I left the hospital. The pharmacy had even signed up for monthly home deliveries for these medications.

Thankfully, my nausea had subsided, but my head was still pounding. I was not going to let this headache ruin my day though. I was going home...with new lungs! A day I had dreamed about for so long. I felt emotionally ready to go home; as if I could make it on my own now, without the call button and a nurse just a hop, skip and a jump away. I could do this.

I let the excitement of seeing my daughter and sleeping in my own bed fill me up. The thought of being able to sleep through the night without any nurses waking me made me practically jump out of that bed! A night full of rest sounded like a pure dream. I was expected back the next two days for rehabilitation so I wouldn't be gone for long. About sixteen hours later to be exact.

16
Home Sweet Home

When I got home, I surprised my daughter. When she got off the school bus, she came running and gave me a huge hug! Boy, did I need that! I missed her hugs and cuddles so much. It was a great reminder as to why I went through the years of struggle, pain, heartache, and finally, surgery. Now, it was time to fully recover and start working on her bucket list that she made us.

Being at home with new lungs was very startling. The first thing I noticed was how quiet our house was. I was used to the constant humming and turning over of the oxygen concentrator. I was used to the percussion sounds of "The Vest" chest physical therapy. The loud air compressor running on my nebulizer, which gave me my breathing treatments, was the norm.

It was so quiet that it was eerie. I was not used to this life, and I had to learn my new normal. I didn't know what normal was like. Ever since I was little, my house hummed with machines that helped me breathe better. The lack of coughing also made for a huge void in noise. The louder my coughs and machines were, the louder my television or conversations had to be, making for a very noisy atmosphere.

Another strange concept was not having the fifty foot oxygen tube to carry along with me as I traveled throughout the house. I had certain pathways I would take to certain rooms that enabled me to keep the tube from getting twisted and kinked. Now, I could go anywhere I wanted in the house. When I needed to go to our basement, it was no longer a daunting chore. I could walk up and down the stairs as many times as needed, even carrying things. I was so set in my ways before just so I could exist and get through each day.

My husband and daughter had to actually come to find me when they needed me. They could no longer just follow the oxygen tube. We were beyond thrilled to start making plans together as a family. We could travel, go on family hikes, and truly, have hope for a future together. I had survived a life-changing event and now we all had to reteach ourselves how to live. We were no longer tied down by an illness. We could live the way we wanted to. Live the way we had always dreamed of. Live like a normal family.

The first day of pulmonary rehabilitation was the first day of my new life. In rehab, I was nicknamed, "The 1%-er," which I proudly sported every day. My rehab was five days per week for twelve weeks. In addition, I had to do bloodwork to ensure my anti-rejection medication was at the optimal levels in my bloodstream at all times. There was a chest x-ray twice per week to make sure no abnormalities formed. I performed a lung function test once per week where I got to experience the joy of watching my lung function climb. I had never seen my lung function increase.

I saw the transplant doctor every week. I came with a list of questions each time to ensure I remained educated on my new immunosuppressed life. I wanted to follow all the rules to maximize my life expectancy with new lungs. I underwent a bronchoscopy once per month to check for infection and rejection. It was quite a schedule.

I was surprised patients of similar age were also sitting in the waiting room wearing masks. There were five of us who all received double lung transplants within a month of each other and were in pulmonary rehab. I grew to learn each of their stories and transplant experiences. They all had CF just like me, but all of them were from out of town. They had made a huge sacrifice coming to this hospital to have their lung transplant and the twelve weeks of rehab thereafter.

Prior to transplant, CF patients are not allowed close contact with each other due to the possibility of passing along harmful bacteria to each other. It was a new concept to be able to sit and talk to someone with CF. The CF moms sat and chatted with each other while we were in our testings and rehab, which gave them a support group too.

Three days after my release from the hospital, I had a scare. I woke up not being able to lift my left arm. The swelling under my arm on my side had worsened. I immediately called my doctor and went to the emergency room.

As luck would have it, no one was in the emergency room. We walked right in and right to the triage area. After spending all day in the emergency room, the doctors determined the lymph nodes under my arm were swollen. But, there was not enough fluid to be drained. With time, the swelling and pain would gradually subside. I was relieved and elated to be heading back home.

On the drive home, we stopped for dinner. It was one of the first times I realized the potential and the ease of my new life. We could stop and eat out at our leisure after being gone from home all day. I wasn't exhausted. I didn't have to push myself and expect repercussions the next day. I didn't have to rush home to do my breathing treatments before I ate. I didn't have to rush home before my oxygen tank ran out. I didn't have to play "beat the clock" anymore. We could park far away from the door of the restaurant. I could walk without a struggle and as far as I needed to. I didn't need to sit down as soon as I walked into the restaurant. I was not out of breath.

This was just thirteen days after I received new lungs, and it was the same day my family also realized how much my life had changed. My mom and dad were in disbelief that I could spend all day away from home, go out to eat, and then come to their house and go up and down the stairs with no difficulty. My husband did not feel rushed to get me home before my oxygen ran out or exhaustion set in on me. It was truly amazing for them to witness.

It was time to share my story. I wanted to share with others just how important organ donation is. I was honored to do a follow-up story on television increasing lung transplant awareness a second time. I wanted people to see the impact organ donation can have on a whole family.

I also shared my story at church through a video. I imagined and anticipated the physical obstacles I would need to achieve when receiving a transplant, but I did not anticipate the spiritual responsibility and debt I felt. I needed to tell others what God had done for me and how my prayers were answered.

One man expressed his immense gratitude for me sharing my story. It was life-saving for him. He did not want to come to church that day, but he felt a pull to attend. He had planned to commit suicide the following Thursday. He watched my video story and saw how my life was a constant battle and in the end, God was faithful. After hearing my story, he changed his mind and decided to keep fighting. He was no longer going to commit suicide. One life saved!

The one question on everyone's mind was, "What now?" For as long as I could remember, I longed for the transplant, but now, I had no future plans. My short term plan was always to get a transplant, and there was no long term plan. I never looked past that huge obstacle. What *would* I do now?

I felt a little lost in my new life and was not sure how to navigate through this uncharted territory. I was fearful the shoe would drop at any moment or I would wake up from a dream. Things were just going too well for me, for my whole family. I was used to a constant battle with illness and frequent hospitalizations that I simply was not used to an easy road.

My first plan of action was to fulfill my daughter's bucket list. She filled her list with items we could not do before, such as ride bikes, jump on the trampoline, go on vacation, and walk the dog. One morning, we were playing tag at the bus stop, and I ran to tag her. I caught up to her and she exclaimed, "I forgot you can run now!" She always won tag and hide-and-seek before. The endless possibilities of new adventures with her were so heartwarming.

My future is so bright, and it is time to start living life to the fullest.

Epilogue

I am almost two years post-transplant and happy to say "I am rejection-free!" Praise God! I am thirty-four years old and have slowly found my way in my new life. I am working, traveling with my family, and trying to give back. My daughter is now nine years old. She has gone through so much, and I am so proud of the compassionate, kind person that she is. We have completed all of the items on Molly's bucket list and thoroughly enjoyed marking each item off the list. My family calls me "The Energizer Bunny." At times, I have to remember to reign myself in and still prioritize my life for those most important to me. My journey taught me that.

It has been incredible to see what has came to fruition for my entire family since my transplant. My transplant changed all of our lives. Each of us has developed a new passion, pastime, or charity to volunteer with. My health is no longer a huge time constraint or emotional drain on anyone. One door closed and a new window opened.

I owe so much to all of my doctors, nurses, and care teams that I have had over many years of care. I am still in contact with all of them, and I really hope they understand the true gift they gave me by providing excellent care and getting me to that transplant. My care teams and parents are the reason I surpassed the statistic I was given at birth of only living to eighteen years old.

I am so incredibly humbled, awestruck, and grateful for the two miracles God has given me: my daughter and my new lungs. My organ donor was a female who was sixty-seven years old. I pray that my donor's family is at peace knowing they saved my life and also gave me a whole new life. I have the opportunity to see my daughter grow up and tell others exactly what God has done in my life because of her choice to donate her organs. My church family calls me, "A Celebrity for God."

While my new lungs now work incredibly, I still have CF in the rest of my body and always will. Fortunately, my new lungs will never develop the CF. There will always be a chance of rejection though. Transplant is not a cure, and I am facing a 50% survival rate at five years. Chronic rejection is inevitable for lung transplant patients. It is just a matter of when. I do not know how long my perfect new lungs will last, but I am choosing to trust God and not take a single day for granted.

My life with CF and transplant journey have changed the way I live my life. I do not procrastinate and I truly live in the moment. My journey has made me who I am today. My sister believes our close knit family is because of my CF and transplant struggles.

Today, I continue to make memories with my family and plan for our future. I am helping my daughter pursue her dream of horses and support my husband's career goals and passions. I am a living, breathing, testament to God's faithfulness and His miracles. I am breathing deep every day.

"With men this is impossible; but with God all are things are possible." Matthew 19:26

Molly's Bucket List

*M*y daughter made a bucket list for us to accomplish together after I received my new lungs.

The simple pleasures in life are the most important.

1 ripe Bikes together
2 We x Play With Buddy
3 we can Go to the Lake
4 we can Go to the creek
5 Go to mimi and PaPa's.
6 Go on vacation,
7 jump on the trampoline

Scriptures for Your Struggles

*I*t took me thirty years before I realized that I had a true reference for living right at my fingertips—the Bible. My bible sat in my nightstand collecting dust for years. I did not pick up and truly study the Bible until my life depended on it, and I had nowhere to turn. No one truly understood what I was feeling and how scared I was. Life is messy, hard, and full of struggles, but I hope these scriptures can give you some comfort in whatever trials you are facing.

Cast all your anxiety on him because he cares for you.
1 Peter 5:7

The Lord will fight for you, and you have only to be still.
Exodus 14:14

He gives power to the faint, and to him who has no might he increases strength.
Isaiah 40:29

Trust in the Lord with all your heart, and do not lean on your own understanding.

Proverbs 3:5

I can do all this through him who gives me strength.

Philippians 4:13

Consider it pure joy, my brothers and sisters, whenever you face trials of many kinds, because you know that the testing of your faith produces perseverance.

James 1: 2-3

Don't be afraid, for I am with you. Don't be discouraged, for I am your God. I will strengthen you and help you. I will hold you up with my victorious right hand.

Isaiah 41:10

Be strong and courageous. Do not fear or be in dread of them, for it is the LORD your God who goes with you. He will not leave you or forsake you.

Deuteronomy 31:6

Blessed is the one who perseveres under trial because, having stood the test, that person will receive the crown of life that the Lord has promised to those who love him.

James 1:12

Not only so, but we also glory in our sufferings, because we know that suffering produces perseverance; perseverance, character; and character, hope.

Romans 5: 3-4

When the righteous cry for help, the Lord hears and delivers them out of all their troubles. The Lord is near to the brokenhearted and saves the crushed in spirit.

Psalm 34: 17-18

Don't worry about anything; instead, pray about everything. Tell God what you need, and thank him for all he has done. Then you will experience God's peace, which exceeds anything we can understand.

Philippians 4: 6-7

For I know the plans I have for you, says the Lord. They are plans for good and not for disaster, to give you a future and a hope. In those days when you pray, I will listen.

Jeremiah 29: 11

Come to me, all of you who are weary and carry heavy burdens, and I will give you rest.

Matthew 11: 29

But blessed are those who trust in the Lord and have made the Lord their hope and confidence. They are like trees planted along a riverbank, with roots that reach deep into the water. Such trees are not bothered by the heat or worried by long months of drought. Their leaves stay green, and they never stop producing fruit.

Jeremiah 17: 7-8

Appendix I
Resources for Cystic Fibrosis Patients and Families

- *Cystic Fibrosis Foundation- They are a non-profit organization and can provide a great wealth of useful information. This foundation is the perfect go-to website for any information needed for CF patients and caregivers. There are 70 chapters across the country and are easily accessible.*

  http://www.cff.org

- *Boomer Esiason Foundation- A non-profit organization that was founded by a father with a child who has Cystic Fibrosis. It raises awareness of Cystic Fibrosis through various programs, events, and supporting research to find a cure.*

  http://www.esiason.org

- *Cystic Fibrosis Research Inc. (CFRI)- This non-profit organization spreads awareness of Cystic Fibrosis with an emphasis on research.*

  http://www.cfri.org

- *Claire's Place Foundation- A non-profit organization that was founded by a Cystic Fibrosis patient. Its mission is to provide Cystic Fibrosis patients and families with financial and emotional support.*

  http://www.clairesplacefoundation.org

- *Genentech Access Solutions- Genentech is the producer of Pulmozyme. Pulmozyme is a daily medication used by Cystic Fibrosis patients, and Genentech offers payment assistance programs for Genentech medications.*

  http://www.genentech-access.com

Appendix II
Resources for Transplant Patients and Families

- *Transplant Living- A helpful website run by the United Network of Organ Sharing (UNOS) that is informational, educational, and supportive for patients and families. There is also a full list of organizations that provide financial aid for transplant patients.*

  https://transplantliving.org

- *Organ Donation- Run by the U.S. Department of Health and Human Services and the Donate Life campaign, these websites are the official sites to sign up as an organ donor along with statistics and personal transplant stories.*

http://www.organdonor.gov

http://www.registerme.org

- *United Network for Organ Sharing (UNOS)- This is the non-profit organization that is in charge of the transplant waiting list. On their website, you can find how they match organs, prioritize patients who are waiting, and personal stories.*

https://unos.org

- *Organ Procurement and Transplantation Network (OPTN)- This organization is run under the U.S. Department of Health and Human Services, and is contracted with UNOS. Their website offers educational resources, such as allocation processes and systems that are in place, along with professional education, news, and resources.*

http://optn.transplant.hrsa.gov

- *American Transplant Foundation- A non-profit organization offering emotional support through mentoring, financial assistance to patients, and education, to everyone regardless of their legal status.*

http://www.americantransplantfoundation.org

About the Author

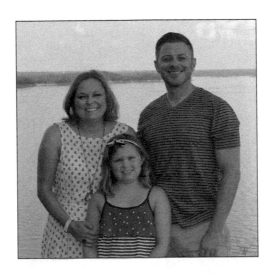

*K*elly was born with Cystic Fibrosis and continues to fight this fatal disease every day. She underwent a double lung transplant in 2017 and faces new challenges with post-transplant life. Kelly has a Masters in Social Work degree and previously worked with end-stage kidney disease patients. Currently, Kelly owns a small business toy shop called "Miss Sunshine's Toy Shoppe," and a mobile notary business. Kelly received the "Hero of Hope Award," which is a national award given *to Cystic Fibrosis patients for their strength, courage, positive attitude, diligence in self-care, and a "special spark." Kelly was also featured on KMOV news television for her miraculous story pre- and post-transplant, and highlighted in a testimonial story at Morning Star Church in Dardenne Prairie, Missouri. She enjoys movies, traveling, being active, and making memories with her family. Kelly lives in Defiance, Missouri with her husband and daughter.*

Organg Donation

*There are **114,590** men, women, and children waiting for a transplant.*
*Every **10** minutes another person is added to the transplant wait list.*
***20** people die each day waiting for a transplant.*
*Only **3** in **1,000** people die in a way that allows for organ donation.*

1 ORGAN DONOR CAN SAVE 8 LIVES

Please sign up to be an organ donor at:
http://www.registerme.org

*Transplantation Facts taken from:
http://www.organdonor.gov and http://www.unos.org

You are making a Difference!

A portion of every book purchased will be donated to:

Cystic Fibrosis Foundation & Mid-America Transplant

Together we can continue to work towards a cure for CF and raise awareness about the importance of organ donation.

CPSIA information can be obtained
at www.ICGtesting.com
Printed in the USA
FSHW010730010219
55389FS